Back from the Edge

To Albie and Amelie, being your daddy is the proudest thing in my life. You are bright, kind, funny and compassionate, and I feel so lucky that you are my children. All I ever want is you to feel my love and feel the freedom to fly in this world. This book is dedicated to you because it represents where we are now. I love you with all that I have and always will. x

Back from the Edge

Mental Health and Addiction in Sport

Luke Sutton

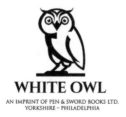

WHITE OWL
AN IMPRINT OF PEN & SWORD BOOKS LTD.
YORKSHIRE - PHILADELPHIA

First published in Great Britain in 2019 and reprinted in 2020 by
Pen & Sword White Owl
An imprint of
Pen & Sword Books Ltd
Yorkshire - Philadelphia

Copyright © Luke Sutton, 2019, 2020

ISBN 978 1 5267 6754 7

Typeset in INDIA by IMPEC eSolutions
Printed and bound in England by TJ International Ltd.

Pen & Sword Books Ltd incorporates the Imprints of Pen & Sword Books
Archaeology, Atlas, Aviation, Battleground, Discovery, Family History,
History, Maritime, Military, Naval, Politics, Railways, Select, Transport,
True Crime, Fiction, Frontline Books, Leo Cooper, Praetorian Press,
Seaforth Publishing, Wharncliffe and White Owl.

For a complete list of Pen & Sword titles please contact

PEN & SWORD BOOKS LIMITED
47 Church Street, Barnsley, South Yorkshire, S70 2AS, England
E-mail: enquiries@pen-and-sword.co.uk
Website: www.pen-and-sword.co.uk

or

PEN AND SWORD BOOKS
1950 Lawrence Rd, Havertown, PA 19083, USA
E-mail: uspen-and-sword@casematepublishers.com
Website: www.penandswordbooks.com

Contents

Chapter 1

Saturday, 14 October 2011.
I was 35 years old. A professional cricketer for the last seventeen years, a captain, a business owner, a respected leader, a father, a husband and I guess what some considered a 'success'. And yet, here I was, sat on my bed, staring out the window at a grass bank, tears pouring down my face, in a place some describe as a 'rehabilitation centre' and others, more honestly, call an 'acute psychiatric hospital'.

Where did it start and finish for me to end up here?

Again, and again and again, it was all I kept saying in my head. I was sobbing. I was really sobbing. Uncontrollably sobbing like I did as a young boy. Sobbing a deep pain of loneliness and confusion. I was completely fucked.

On the outside, I had much more to lose, certainly materially, but on the inside, something had snapped in me. I had so little clarity, my brain was cloudy and confused, but what clarity I did have told me three things:

I was lonely. Desperately lonely.

I was broken.

And nothing would ever be the same.

***

Ten days earlier …

It was my thirty-fifth birthday and the beginning of the end of a very long and painful process for me. Don't get me wrong, I was already completely off the rails at this point, but it seemed like this ten-day run-in was the jumping-off point.

Jimmy and Daniella Anderson had invited me to birthday drinks at their house, and then we were 'out'. The truth is that I had been 'out' for a month. By this time I had already moved out of the family home and was living in an apartment on my own. It was better that way, I thought. People needed to leave me alone and let me just get on with the way I wanted to live my life. That would definitely be better. For starters, it was everyone else's fault that I had all this pressure and shit to deal with. If people would just leave me alone, it would be better, *I* would be better. That's what I thought.

That night my anxiety was off the charts. It hadn't been good for a long time, but this was really different. I had this horrific feeling of doom. I just couldn't shake it. Looking back, in my heart I knew then that I was fucked. It was all coming to a head.

I have never had the steadiest of hands, but I could always rely on a few drinks to level me out. Not this night. We started with champagne, the paradox of this elegance not lost on me. Two or three glasses and that should settle me – not this time. My shaking, my sweating, my nervousness, my involuntary movements; I was all over the place. I couldn't drink the champagne fast enough, but it wasn't working. I couldn't actually stand in the same place for very long or even try to hold a conversation. I needed to be 'out'.

That night out was like many others. I was working full time to try to show people how successful, smart and together I was, and deep down I was falling apart. I knew that others would go to bed that night at some time, but I wouldn't. I would keep going into the darkest hours, where I felt the most comfortable. The great irony was that I was desperately lonely and yet all I wanted was to be alone. In my darkest moments during that night, I found the aloneness I craved. Well, that's what I thought.

The next nine days followed a similar pattern. I would drink for as long as I could, pass out for a few hours and wake up with this horrific feeling of anxiety and doom. It genuinely seemed logical to me that the first thing I would do on awakening would be to drink again. Just a couple of drinks and I would settle and could crack on with the day! What had set in and I was desperately trying to hide from everyone – no one more so than myself – was that I had become a twenty-four-hour drinker. It was there right in front of me but all I could see was that anyone would drink like this if they had my problems.

There was a trip to London during these few days, which ended with me being stuck in the bar at Euston station, crippled by anxiety and unable to get myself on a train back up north. I kept looking at the departures board but couldn't face the prospect of actually getting on to a train. It sounds ridiculous but, in my mind, it was very real. The possibility of choosing a train to get on to, and then actually getting on it, was too much for me. So, I just sat in the station bar ordering two pints at a time, crying, laughing, and utterly delirious with tiredness and drunkenness. If only I could get rid of this anxiety, then I could get back to functioning on some sort of level. But my old friend, the booze, was letting me down in this time of need.

Remarkably, I bumped into Glen and Kerry Chapple at Euston as they were returning from Lancashire CCC's trip to Buckingham Palace for their County Championship win that year. A light was truly shining on me that day because without them, I wouldn't have been able to get on a train, and who knows where I would have ended up? With some persuasion, and a bit of humour, they got me on the train and back I went up north.

I didn't know where all this was heading. To be honest, I had given up. I just didn't care any more. I didn't want to live but I didn't have the guts to kill myself. That was me right then and there.

***

Twenty-four hours earlier …

I woke up in a chair in the Chapples' kitchen. They had let me stay there the night before. I was still fully clothed, with a whisky in front of me. I was obviously still drunk but that was hardly big news at that time. Somehow, I had remembered that my daughter needed to go to hospital that day.

Amelie had recently been diagnosed with type 1 diabetes, which had been hugely traumatic, and this was a consultation with the relevant doctor. It goes without saying that I had been close to useless for my then wife and daughter throughout that time. In some ways it was a miracle that I remembered the appointment. The house was only a walk away. So I finished off my whisky, picked myself up and walked back to the house. Insanely, this all seemed completely normal to me. Sure, I wasn't at my best, but it didn't even cross my mind that I might just look like a park bench drunk.

I strolled into the house and gave the kids big cuddles. I was shaking a lot when I picked them up, but they seemed happy to see me and obviously didn't really know what the stench of alcohol was. I was there with ten minutes to spare to leave for hospital ... virtually a model father and partner.

'You're not coming to hospital, Luke.'

'Why?'

'Because you're drunk, Luke ...'

The absolute fucking cheek of my then wife, Jude! Sure, I was a bit wobbly, but the kids were happy I was there, and I *was* actually there, so what was the problem? Yup, that was me back then.

I didn't go to hospital. Jude got the kids into the car quickly and drove off before I could physically challenge that decision. It wasn't really a contest. I burst into tears and that overwhelming feeling of doom was back in the pit of my stomach. I knew I was nearing the end of whatever journey I was on. I just wanted someone or something to help me. I made some pathetic calls to friends and whaled at them incoherently down the phone. Nothing could help me and so there was only one thing to do ...

Alcohol. Yes, it was 8.45 am but a couple of drinks would settle me. I did have the presence of mind to wonder how I could hide this from Jude. It was her alcohol after all, and God forbid that she find out I'd been drinking at this time of the day. Red wine was the answer. A couple of reasons – it was strong, and the bottle was dark. I could unscrew the top, have a glass or two and then place the bottle back on the rack, and at first glance no one would know that it wasn't full. Genius!

So, there I was, sat on the kitchen floor, crying and drinking red wine … at 8.45 am, when I should have been at the hospital supporting my daughter. That was me.

I did pick myself up, though. And obviously walked to a bar in Altrincham. I drive past that bar on a regular basis nowadays and always give it a wry smile. It's a dive and it was perfect for me on that day. Firstly, it opened early enough but it also matched what I had become. Looking back, it felt like I was there for ten minutes, but I know now I was there for nearly six hours. I just couldn't stop drinking. I was absolutely desperate. I didn't talk to anyone in the bar and had spells of crying followed by spells of deep drunken bliss. I had no plan. Just one drink after another.

I did my customary calls to a couple of friends in which I was basically asking for help. What kind of help, I had no idea. On this day, these calls pushed the alarm bells to another level and my friends felt they needed to act. All of a sudden, two of my closest teammates, Glen Chapple and Mark Chilton, walked into the bar and sat down with me. Mark is someone I have known since I was 12 years old and I respect him hugely. Glen is a really good friend whom I had grown closer to during my time at Lancashire CCC.

Jimmy and Daniella Anderson and Glen and Kerry Chapple have always been incredible friends to me, and right at that moment, they were trying to help. I don't think anyone actually knew what to do with me. I didn't know at this point that Kerry had gone ahead and rung The Priory to book me an appointment. I will be eternally grateful to them all.

I was really happy to see Glen and Mark but the first thing I said was that they should not try to make me leave the bar. I actually muttered that I would fight them if they tried, which would have made for a hilarious scene. They were incredible and just sat with me. They didn't rush me even though I'm sure they were pretty alarmed by the state I was in. We talked, I cried, and obviously I drank more. I don't know how long we were sat there but they eventually persuaded me to go back to Glen's house under the agreement that I could continue drinking.

I don't remember travelling to Glen's house, but I do remember being there. I sat outside drinking whisky. Suddenly my dad walked in. It was absolutely devastating. I knew how I looked. Knowing that my dad could see me like this was awful. He was clearly distressed too. He sat with me and asked me to go back to my apartment with him. After some time, I agreed.

It was at this time that The Priory was first mentioned to me and I just laughed about it.

What can they do to help me?

I didn't even know what was wrong with me but was happy to cast aspersions over who could and couldn't help me. I don't remember much from then on other than arriving back at my apartment and my mum was also there. It was horrific. Their 35-year old son was a mess and I couldn't hide it. If that shame was bad, the night in the apartment was horrendous. They obviously wouldn't let me drink, and a combination of alcohol withdrawal and sleep deprivation made the night a living nightmare. I had visions of monsters in the room and drifted in and out of sleep. As a boy, I used to have this reccurring dream that orange (no idea why that colour) monsters were climbing up my walls. I was right back there. A little boy. Terrified and so lonely.

The next morning, I literally begged them to take me to The Priory. I had no idea what was wrong, but I knew I needed help.

***

Forty-five minutes earlier …

My devastated mum and dad had been checking in their adult child to this centre. I can't imagine how hard that was for them. I remember little of it all, but I do recall having my medical check-in with a tall, bald, Scottish man called Dennis. He was a pleasant man, just doing the job he had done thousands of times before with people from all walks of life who had got themselves into a similar state as me.

Blood pressure.

Heart rate.

Temperature.

'When was the last time you drank alcohol?'

'What was it and how much?'

'Have you taken any drugs?' …

'If I don't feel better in forty-eight hours then I'm coming back to fucking see you!'

That's all I could say to Dennis. That was me. I'm the one checking in to an acute psychiatric hospital and that's all I could say to this lovely man. And that really was me. Huge ego, already looking to pin the blame on others, and yet I was breaking into little pieces.

***

Sitting on my bed in The Priory was the start of a huge process for me, but I didn't know that then. I was just scared and lonely. But strangely, I will never forget the tremendous feeling of relief I had on that day.

The game is up.

I was actually relieved that I could stop pretending that everything was OK. Everything was not fucking OK. Everything was really wrong. It was such hard work pretending to everyone that I had everything under control. It was like a full-time job. I knew this moment was a tipping point and I could or should no longer pretend.

I guess it was my first moment of letting go. Letting go of trying to be someone I thought everyone wanted. I had very little clarity at this point. I didn't even know where to start or what to do, but I did have this feeling of relief.

I needed life to stop because I just couldn't cope. Sitting in The Priory, locked away, I was actually safe. No calls, no emails, no drinking, no pretending, no nothing. Just me.

However, the relief was not matched by hope. I had no hope. It was just darkness in my mind. It wasn't that I had become someone I didn't want to be; I didn't actually know who I was. I felt like a wafer-thin piece of paper that had been ripped into a million pieces. They were all jumbled up, so how on earth was anyone going to be able to put this all back together? I definitely couldn't.

I was broken.
Where did it start and finish for me to end up here?

***

I really have so much to tell you.

My story is no more or less important than anyone else's, but it is an opportunity to share my experience in one go. It's not a story of mental health issues, addiction issues or professional sport issues; it is a story of all of them wrapped into one.

The overwhelming feeling for me during my darkest times was loneliness. I don't want anyone to ever feel like that, so I guess this book is a way to reach out to others. For a long time, I didn't think I should write this book, but I guess the question in the end for me was, *why not?* I couldn't find a good enough reason to not do it.

I'm not ashamed about my journey, although I wish I hadn't done some of the things I have. I also appreciate that they needed to happen for me to find another way to live my life. People will make their judgements ... but they always have, and that's OK. I know what I am now and there is no power in that judgement.

I want to live a life of meaning and substance that my loved ones, particularly my children, can be proud of. I hope this book can also make them proud.

Chapter 2

From my early twenties, I knew that alcohol was an issue for me. It was a dark secret that I tried to keep from everyone – no one more so than myself.

It was nothing to do with the quantity or frequency that I drank; it was the impact it had on me. I'm not here to tell anyone what is and isn't a problem with alcohol – I just know what a problem it was for me. Many of my tales will be shared by lots of young people and other professional sportspeople who don't end up with the difficulties that I did, but it was enough for me.

I thought I had found myself with alcohol, but I actually completely lost myself. I describe this journey as spiralling around an ever-decreasing circle. To start with, it is moving so slowly you don't even know that it is happening, but gradually, over time, you slide further down, and the circle gets tighter and the speed of the journey increases. You certainly know about it then.

***

Dermot Reeve was my first ever county head coach at Somerset CCC, and on a cricket level, he was utterly inspiring. He had an extraordinary cricket brain and was ahead of his time in many ways. I loved working with him and those early years with him definitely shaped my entire career. Dermot has had his own well-documented issues with drugs and I believe he and I shared a persona within cricket that eventually led to our difficulties. My early days at Somerset CCC were very much about finding this persona and believing I had 'arrived'!

I stepped into professional cricket pretty much straight from school, and the environment was very much 'Work hard, play hard'. I guess it was what we call 'old school'. An element of that still exists today but nowhere near to the same extent. My first second team away match with Somerset CCC was at Yorkshire CCC and as we arrived at the hotel the night before, all the chat was about what bars and clubs we were going to that night in Leeds. This wasn't a shock to anyone; it was just the way it was.

Although I had come from privileged schooling at Millfield School and was very confident in a number of ways, I was desperate for affirmation and to find where I 'fitted in'. It sounds crazy because people imagine professional sportspeople all to be super confident, and in some ways we are, but underneath the surface can lie much insecurity. It was not difficult to persuade me to hit the town; I just wanted to be one of the lads and, in truth, I enjoyed the bars and clubs, as most young people do.

True to form, we had a big night. A 4.00 am finish, followed by a 7.30 am wake-up for breakfast. Some lads were able to control themselves to a degree, but I couldn't. If I started, then it would only be big. What I realised very early on was that the key was how I backed it up the next morning. And the old school mentality was very much that it didn't matter what you did the night before as long as you were on top form the next day. So probably through a mixture of self-preservation instinct and determination, I always made sure I was on peak form the next day, even if I was dying inside.

This early 'Work hard, play hard' mentality really worked for me. It was the persona that made me believe that I had arrived in the world. I didn't necessarily go drinking as much as some people, but when I did it was huge. On the flip side, when I worked hard it was with an equal level of intensity. You almost develop a warrior mentality within this persona, which teammates admire. I was a player with limited ability, so this determination to do everything to an extreme worked for me for nearly twenty years in the game. I genuinely thought I had found myself. I was good at drinking and I was good at working hard, and everyone seemed happy with me for it. That's what mattered to me most at that time, so all was good.

I actually believed I had a method to cricket and life. It was all about punishment and reward. My reward for working extremely hard was going out partying equally hard; and my punishment for excessive drinking was to work with ferocious intensity. No one had an issue with it and it seemed to help position me as a leader in most teams I played in. I am a Libran and used to tell people that it was my balance in life. My imbalance was my balance! Looking back, there was some logic within all this madness.

Many people will read this who share the same mentality and experience and not have the difficulties I have had. But for me, it was the start of the falling apart of the persona I had built up for myself. I was travelling towards the centre of my ever-decreasing circle and had no idea it was happening.

After my first season at Somerset, I went on an end-of-season golf trip to Marbella with Dermot and a few others. One of the people on the trip was Jason Kerr, now the Somerset head coach and my then best friend. I obviously wasn't going for the golf! This trip was perfect for me: away from home and free to get into drinking difficulties without too much fuss. Plus, cricket had ended for the summer. It proved to be the trip when I got my first inclination that drinking was different for me.

Jason will admit that he always loved a night out, but he could balance things far better than I could. On that trip, I completely ran out of money. And I mean completely ran out. No cash, no cards … nothing. We had two nights left and this was a big problem. If you are someone who can't stop drinking on a night out, then you really can't have a limit on the money you have access to. Jason was happy to lend me some, but I knew it would never be enough. The prospect of having to control my drinking or, even worse, not drink at all was just too much for me. I was crippled by insecurities, and having to try to talk to girls, or anyone, for that matter, on a night out was virtually impossible without alcohol. I got in a complete panic about it. I borrowed the money from Jason and went through it fast. I had to go back to him for more and was virtually begging. It was the frenzy that I was in that was the most startling thing. It prompted Jason to question what was going on with my drinking. I didn't admit it to him then but I knew that, for me, drinking was something different than it was for most other people.

Without it, I felt completely lost as a person.

***

I spent three winters playing Grade Cricket in Sydney and had some really happy times there. The cricket was brilliantly hard, and I learnt so much about myself as a player. Sydney was also the place that I discovered twenty-four-hour drinking. At that time in England, nightclubs shut at around 2.00 am and that was it. In Sydney, it never stopped. On my first trip there I travelled and lived with Andrew Strauss. We were good friends at university and flew off to Australia together wide-eyed and as wet behind the ears as you could imagine.

Our first night there was a nondescript Tuesday evening and there was never a reason to go home. I still remember drunkenly walking the streets of Kings Cross at 8.30 am as people were off to work. The strange thing about Sydney was that it was a hugely sociable place for me, but it was also the place I started drinking on my own in the dead of night. As everyone headed home for the night, I would head to a bar on my own. And these weren't high-class bars. You basically spoke to the barman and that was it. It was a really strange habit to get into, but I found something comforting about drinking in a dead-end bar with people who had no expectations of me. It was like I could escape the pressure I placed on myself to be someone. The internal battles I constantly had with myself were exhausting and in the early hours, when I was in a drunken bliss, I found escape. Escape from me.

After the 2002/03 New Year's Eve in Sydney, I decided not to drink at all until the last day of Derbyshire CCC's preseason tour to Portugal in late March. I had never trained so hard, and switched my intensity to my weight and fitness. I was weighing myself fifteen to twenty times a day and was utterly obsessed with the number on the scales. I wanted to get to 80kg and then when I did, it wasn't enough.

Then I wanted 78kg, and the pattern started again. Looking back, all of it was odd behaviour, but it is who I thought I was. I believed that I found happiness in obsession and achievement.

I duly went on the preseason tour to Portugal with Derbyshire CCC and was on really good form. From a performance point of view, it couldn't have gone better, but I also knew that the last night of the tour was coming and was equally ready for it!

I don't really know where to begin with it, to be honest. I started the evening off by punching my good friend Lian Wharton in the face for no particular reason. I had actually been staying with him and his parents before the tour. I then blacked out for four hours before waking up, face down, in the car park of the resort we were in. And when I say 'blacked out', I don't mean passed out unconscious, I mean I was awake and moving around the area but have zero memory of it. I am highlighting this one incident, but the truth is that I used to black out a lot while drinking.

We had an early morning flight home and I was blind drunk on the bus and then on the plane. In essence, this isn't that big a deal and this does tend to happen to young men. I was 27 years old at the time and had just completed an excellent preseason tour for my county team. In fact, I was just about to embark on the most successful season of my career to date. So all was not that bad; in fact, all was good. Well, that is what I would tell myself.

But these sorts of incidents would eat away at me. I hadn't drunk for three months and yet there was no control when I did, there was no off button, and I behaved in a way that I was ashamed of. I would play the game and laugh with the lads on the bus, but underneath the surface I was just pushing down shame. And the horrible reality is that I was doing this again and again and again. My ever-decreasing circle.

If those twenty-four hours were bad, it was nothing compared to the twenty-four hours to come. We arrived back from Portugal that evening and were straight into training the next day. Remember my 'punishment and reward' method to cricket and life? Well, the following morning was a prime time to punish myself for the excesses in Portugal. I embarked on a brutal few hours of wicket-keeping drills.

I even wore extra training clothing to increase how much I sweated. I very nearly passed out a number of times. What was I trying to get rid of? Sweat or shame? I knew the truth.

It was a huge training session for me that I had completely instigated myself. No coach asked me to do it, but I needed to do it to repent for Portugal. I was basically purging, and I did this all the time. This 'method' is what helped coaches and teammates see me as a model professional. OK, I had the odd blowout, but this I more than made up for with my training. People admired me for the intensity I brought to training but sadly there was more to it than just trying to be a good pro. I was punishing myself.

I finished training about 3.00 pm and, after a shower, met our then head coach, Adrian Pearson, for a coffee. He wanted to chat about the season ahead and my role within it. I loved Adrian as a person and a coach but during the meeting I started to feel seriously ill. Eventually I had to excuse myself and went back to the apartment I had just bought. The apartment was brand new and basically had a mattress in it and nothing else. The pain in my stomach was excruciating. To this day, I have never felt pain like it. It felt like I was being repeatedly stabbed in the stomach and it came in waves every few minutes. It was absolutely horrendous. I lay in the foetal position on my mattress and started vomiting repeatedly. Vomiting temporarily relieved the pain, but it would come again worse than the time before.

I hung in there for about an hour but couldn't take any more and called my great friend Michael Di Venuto, who lived in an apartment above me. He came down and tried to help, but quickly realised he needed assistance and called our physiotherapist, Craig Ranson. Craig was an excellent physio and called an ambulance, and the next thing was, I was in hospital in Derby. No one knew what was wrong with me, but my pain was clear for all to see.

I was administered morphine and the relief was extraordinary. As a wicketkeeper, pain is not an unusual experience, but there were times during that episode when I didn't think I could take any more. I stayed at the hospital that night and managed to mostly sleep through. The following morning, the doctors wanted to do some blood tests to understand what was wrong with me. The pain and vomiting had stopped but my main concern was being let out of hospital so I would be ready to play in the first game of the season versus Glamorgan CCC.

After the blood tests results came back a doctor came to see me to discuss what they had found.

'The results show that there are trace amounts of an enzyme that would indicate you have pancreatitis.'

'What's pancreatitis?'

'It's basically a disease in which the pancreas becomes inflamed. It can be very serious.'

'How has this happened?'

'There are a number of ways, but do you drink alcohol a lot?'

'What? I haven't drunk for three months and just had one big night in Portugal!'

'Well, it is just trace amounts, but this is serious. You can die from pancreatitis and I would suggest you don't drink alcohol again.'

'Drink again? What … ever?'

'I think that would be wise.'

The information I was receiving was mind-blowing on a number of levels. I was 27 years old, a professional cricketer, fitter than I had ever been, had not drunk for three months bar one night, and was now being told I might have pancreatitis and should never drink alcohol again.

How on earth was I going to live my life? I had a method. Punishment and reward! Drinking was a big part of my persona; what would I do now? It was really daunting. My parents came to see me, and we all agreed that I should stop drinking. In my eyes, it was more like I would *try* to stop drinking. A subtle but important difference.

I started that season brilliantly with back-to-back centuries in the first two County Championship matches. My form continued, and it felt like my career was moving on to another level. The 2003 season was definitely huge for me. I did stop drinking for the first six weeks of the season and Jason Kerr even commented to me that maybe that was helping my form. I sort of agreed with him but the challenge I faced was that I still had to live my life and had no pressure outlet for the way I operated. I found it so tough.

I had a night out in Derby and tried not drinking. It was a disaster. I couldn't cope with my anxiety and had no alcohol to help me. I sweated profusely and just wanted to hide. In the end, I cracked and started drinking. Again, it wasn't all the time, but it was hugely excessive levels when I did. I didn't get the stomach pain again, so I just cracked on.

Who knows what happened to me when I went to hospital, but it was clearly a warning sign on the pressure I was putting on my body with the extremities of my behaviour. It was a warning I listened to and discarded quickly because I had to get on with coping with life, and it didn't fit with that. I never went for follow-up checks because I didn't want to know. I didn't want anything to get in the way of how I needed to live my life. I repeat: how I *needed* to live my life. It was a need, and I knew no other way.

***

My ever-decreasing circle was certainly moving, and I didn't know about it or, more truthfully, I didn't want to know about it. I was being successful, and people seemed to like me. That was all that mattered to me at that time. What I thought about myself didn't matter. Or so I believed.

2003 and 2004 would prove to be defining years in my life. If 2003 was eventful, it was purely a warm-up for 2004. What was to come was something I was nowhere near able to cope with.

Chapter 3

I was once told by a grief therapist that your mind takes photos of particularly traumatic moments in your life and that is why your memory can be so clear from that particular time. I know that is true because I can remember every single detail of when I found out Nia had died.

***

Nia and I started seeing each other halfway through 2003. We had been really good friends but then it developed into something more. She was a beautiful spirit on the earth, with a kind and loving soul that genuinely cared for people. And people loved Nia. She was fun, adventurous, mischievous and hugely creative. Nia would befriend a tramp in the street and invite him round for tea and biscuits, and later that day look stunningly glamorous on a night out. She could chat to the gentry and then dance on tables. She was a real-life princess to anyone who came in contact with her.

Nia calmed me. I was so insecure about so much and she gave me belief that I was a good person. She gave me confidence in so many ways. She loved me, and I loved her. It was a young love, and we were free and having fun.

In the winter of 2003/04, Nia and I travelled around the east coast of Australia and I was made Derbyshire CCC club captain after Dominic Cork left. It was a really important time for me. My nights out were still always big, but Nia gave some sense of stability to everything. Dave Houghton took over as head coach at the club and I forged a fantastic relationship with him. I have a huge amount of time for Dave.

That season was a really tough one for us as a team. Fortunately, I played pretty well throughout the year and enjoyed the challenge of captaining a young team. Our penultimate game of the season was away at Essex CCC and we were getting thumped. We actually lost late on the third day, which led to a conversation about whether we stayed down that night or travelled back to Derbyshire. I called Nia and she told me to stay down and have a few beers with the lads, and she would stay at her mum and dad's. I really fancied a few drinks that night, but I have deeply regretted that impulse ever since.

I woke up the next morning with a sore head and drove back to Derby. I called Nia throughout the morning at work on her mobile and on the landline. Her mobile never connected and at the Estée Lauder store where she worked, they kept saying she was not there. I didn't know what was going on but didn't think much more about it.

I got back to my apartment, which I now shared with Nia ... and I can picture it as if it were right now. The sun was beaming through the front windows and our cream carpet looked immaculate. I remember looking around the apartment and it was spotless.

Bless her; she has tidied the apartment for when I got home.

I sat at our dining room table blissfully happy despite our loss down at Essex. In two weeks' time, Nia and I were going to Mexico for a big holiday and I had bought an engagement ring. For one of the very few times in my life, I felt relaxed. Life was good. I felt calm.

I called Nia a couple more times but nothing. It was strange, but I was sure all was good. She was probably catching up with one of her friends. As I write this, I can picture the scene as if it was five minutes ago.

Then there was a buzz on the apartment monitor to say someone was at the entrance to the building to see me. For an instant, I thought it was Nia, but she had keys so that was weird. I looked through the video monitor and saw it was her parents, Anne and Emlyn. I got on really well with them and immediately presumed they were coming to see me to ask what my intentions were for the relationship. I felt happy because I could show them the ring and we could talk about it. I buzzed them in, opened the door to the apartment and waited in the corridor for them while holding the door open.

As they walked down the corridor towards me, I knew exactly what had happened. They didn't need to say anything. Their faces said it all.

The next few minutes were a blur. Anne paced around the apartment and tried to explain. Emlyn was absolutely crushed and fell into a chair. He just stared into the air with his mouth wide open.

Nia had been driving to work from her mum and dad's house that morning and lost control around a corner with a steep hillside drop. Her car came off the road and she died.

I fell to my knees and screamed.

I screamed for what felt like an hour and then lay on the floor sobbing. I was engulfed in intense pain and grief. It was horrific. Like I was suffocating and trapped. It seemed like time stood still. The sun was shining so brightly through the windows and the heat of the rays felt like it was burning me. I was paralysed.

I got out the engagement ring to show Anne and Emlyn. I don't know why, but I was just distraught. There were moments of frantic energy and then I would be paralysed again in pain. I just lay on the floor screaming and crying.

In a moment of time, everything changed in my world. And I mean everything.

Nia had died. I trusted in life and it had fucking burnt me. It had fucking burnt me big time.

In a moment, Nia had gone. In a moment, I was a little boy again – scared, lonely and confused.

***

Losing Nia was utterly devastating, and not just for me. She had a very close and loving family and was a very popular local Derbyshire girl. I was also captain of the County Cricket Club so there was a lot of attention around it. The cricket world, as always, were amazing, and the support I received from Dave Houghton, my teammates, the club and the whole game was incredible.

However, I just couldn't cope.

I couldn't cope with the enormity of it all. Everyone was watching me to see if I was OK and how I was handling everything, and it was all from a place of love, but I found the attention too much. Throughout my life I have found it hard to deal with my own internal battles but now I was dealing with the tragedy of losing Nia and everyone watching me. I didn't know what to do or say.

I stayed locked up in my apartment for a few weeks with my family staying and friends visiting. All of Nia's clothes and belongings were there and I insisted that nothing was moved. I would call her voicemail to listen to her voice and pour over old love letters and messages. I was drinking heavily but, in the circumstances, no one would question that.

I had always been someone who was so reliant on the opinion of others for my own security and self-esteem. It was like this, but on steroids now!

Was I crying too much? Too little? Should I play cricket again? What was normal? Did people just like me because of what had happened to me? Did Nia really love me? Did her family really love me?

Everyone was wonderful to me, but it was me I was battling with. The impact of this time has taken me many years to overcome.

The prospect of me being seen as 'weak' or 'defeated' was unbearable. My whole persona was built around 'Work hard, play hard' – be a warrior on and off the field. I couldn't accommodate being crushed; I had to get on with things. I was struggling internally but if I showed anything different, then who was I? I ended up playing out my grief and devastation based on what I thought other people thought of me. It was so damaging, but it was just where I was as a person at that time. Deep down, I didn't know who I was.

I started to get back on with life but there was a crucial decision I made in my head that would ultimately have a devastating impact on me.

Life had burnt me in a really bad way. Up until then, I trusted in the basic way life would work out – you work hard, meet someone, get married and, most importantly, loved ones die when they are old. But the trust had now gone. I made a conscious decision that from then on, I was going to live on my terms. I would take what I wanted from life. It was going to be all about what life could give me, rather than anything that I could give anyone else. I was going to raise the intensity of everything – training, business and partying. Everything would go up more than a notch. And not only that, there became a real darkness about everything I did – my drinking wasn't just about fun and escape; it was now about destruction. It was self-harm.

I didn't know it then, but that mindset would destroy me for years to come.

***

Behind the façade of me being strong and successful in the months after Nia's death, my behaviour was really erratic. It was a pattern that continued on for years and always behind the scenes. I often didn't behave in a way that I was proud of when I was drinking but every time I let someone down, I would just pull out my 'Get Out of Jail Free' card of what had happened to me with Nia. People always cut me slack, but it was appalling of me. Nia was a truly wonderful person, but I used her death to justify some of my behaviour. It was the ultimate shame for me and I would look in the mirror at times and mutter to myself, *People will find out who you really are. You're a fraud.*

I would end up in the wrong places, with the wrong people, and saying things that I should never say. I hated myself for it. It was eating away at my soul but nothing else mattered other than what it looked like from the outside. On the surface I worked hard to look in control, resilient and strong, but underneath I was desperately fragile.

I knew the truth, though, and the shame was the hardest thing about it all. My only answer was to shove it further down in my soul and pretend it wasn't there. It was my only way to survive. I ended up trapped in this existence in which the truth didn't really matter; all that mattered to me was how I appeared to everyone else. The reality of my life was irrelevant. I thought I could live like that but all the time it was eating away at me. It was also exhausting. It was like life was a big play.

It also meant that control was a massive part of my persona. If you are completely dependent on what other people think of you for your own self-worth, then it is really important you control what everyone thinks. Exerting control over those around me became a huge part of my behaviour. I was happy to duck the blame for something and pin it on someone else. I was also happy to fit in with whatever crowd I needed depending on what was important at that time. My values and opinions were irrelevant; in fact, I couldn't even remember what they were. I was just trying to survive but, in the process, I was losing myself.

I do still think of what Nia sees from the heavens. For a long time, I was ashamed of what she could see. My behaviour when drinking was out of control and I wasn't being the best version of myself, but drinking wasn't just important to me, it was everything to me. It was as important to me as training, as it was all part of the same mindset, method … whatever you want to call it. It was the yin and yang of my personality.

So, the answer was never to stop drinking. The answer was to find a way to survive in the world while behaving like that. To this day I have met hundreds of people with addictive behaviour difficulties and they are some of the most resilient people on the earth. They are survivors because life is difficult for them because of their own behaviour, but they have to find a way to get by, and they do for a long time. I was exactly like that.

***

It is really important for me to point something out.

I didn't end up in The Priory because of Nia dying. There were warning signs and progression long before I had even met Nia. Over the years it has been convenient for me to use this tragedy as an excuse, but it didn't happen like that. Nia's death was a monumentally difficult thing to happen in my life and it opened all the vulnerability that existed within me. But it was part of my journey towards falling part, not the start of that journey. I was travelling round my ever-decreasing circle and Nia's death increased the pace of that significantly, but I was already going down.

We have a choice in life to carry forward with us things from our past that then affect our present. Likewise, we have a choice to let them go. For far too long I carried the scars of Nia's death with me and chose not to deal with them. They constantly affected what I was doing and feeling, but make no mistake: that was my choice. I had to learn that there was a better way of finding peace, but it had to come to me breaking into a million pieces for me to be able to do that.

Chapter 4

I can't remember why or when, but I decided to leave my room and sit in the lounge area, which was directly opposite my room in the residential part of The Priory.

There was no one around and I just sat at the big table where some newspapers lay. I didn't take much in from what was in the lounge, but I remember a huge sofa and TV. The thought of having to sit with strangers to watch TV at night was way beyond me at this point.

I wasn't sobbing any more but was feeling incredibly fragile. I felt like I could cry at the smallest thing. I was still overwhelmed with confusion, sadness and deep loneliness. That phrase kept returning in my mind: *Where did it start and finish for me to end up here?*

It also dawned on me that I literally had no idea what I was meant to do there. I either didn't listen when I had been told, or no one had told me. The not listening option was more likely. I felt like I was only able to absorb very basic information.

Looking back, I also realise that I still held on to this arrogance in my mind. I was grateful to be there, to be away from the world, but despite having not yet met anyone, I presumed that I would be different to everyone else there. I wasn't going to be like the down-and-outs in there. I was a professional cricketer, I was a business owner, I was 'something' … I just wasn't like these people. I actually cringe looking back at my attitude. I had completely fallen to pieces and yet here I was placing judgement on who was better than whom. The truth is, I was an arrogant prat.

That's when I first met Lenny.

A small man, mid-thirties, with a shaven head, bounced into the lounge wearing a big puffer jacket. The table I was sat at was near the entrance, so he had virtually gone past me when he did a double take and realised there was a 'newbie' sitting there.

'Alright, lad,' he said in the broadest Scouse accent.

I just nodded back. I was terrified of him. He had a deeply intense stare and immediately got uncomfortably close to me.

'You just got here, lad?'

'Yeah.'

'What programme are you on?'

'I don't know.'

'What's your problem, lad? Is it booze, drugs or something like depression?'

'I've no idea.'

That was the truth; I had no idea why I was there. I knew I needed help but for exactly what, I didn't know. Sure, I had been drinking a lot but if you had my problems, then so would you. I must have been told when I came in, but I hadn't been able to take it in.

'You'll be OK, lad. I got here about a week ago. I'll look out for ya.'

He then leaned down and wrapped his arms around me. He hugged me. Properly hugged me. That was my first of many experiences with Lenny.

Later on, I was to find out that Lenny was a major drug dealer in Liverpool who had got hooked on his own product, heroine, or 'the Brown', as he called it. Being small, Lenny had made an excellent house burglar when he was younger, and then progressed to higher levels of crime throughout the city. Lenny had seen a lot in his life, maybe too much. There was an intensity to him that was intimidating, but there was also something else beneath his eyes. Something softer.

We couldn't have been more different – a salt-of-the-earth gangster versus a silver-spooned, arrogant, professional sportsman. But he didn't care. He had immediately tried to comfort me and make me feel less alone. I sobbed again as he hugged me, and he just kept repeating, 'You'll be alright, lad.'

I had so much more to learn about Lenny, The Priory and, even more so, about myself, but this first interaction was huge for me. A stranger, who knew nothing about me, didn't care about that and just wanted to make me feel better.

I'll never forget Lenny.

***

To put an end to any rumours, The Priory is not some sort of holiday camp for celebrities. If there were Jacuzzis hidden somewhere then I didn't find them. Everything was perfectly fine and functional, but there was no luxury involved. It always made me giggle to hear 'inmates' complain about the pressure of the showers first thing in the morning. We were there to save our lives and were more worried about water pressure.

What The Priory does have are some incredible people. Kind hearts trying to help people like me who have completely lost their way. The day after I met Lenny was my first full day there. I went to breakfast in the canteen and it reminded me of walking into the dining room when I first arrived at Millfield Prep School 'Edgarley Hall' in Glastonbury. Absolutely terrifying.

Lenny did look out for me and introduced me to some other people. Phil arrived the day before me and we all sat together at breakfast. I had never seen someone shake as much as Phil from withdrawals. It was so sad to see, and I helped him cut his breakfast that morning. The saddest part of it was that Phil couldn't really make the connection between his shakes and the withdrawal symptoms from alcohol. I guess it was my first insight into 'denial'. I was still deep in my own denial, but I was happy to observe it in other people.

It turned out I was on 'ATP' – the Addiction Therapy Programme. Lenny explained it to me and I can't say I really agreed with me being on it, but I also didn't really give a shit. I just wanted to get on with some sort of routine there. I also found out I was on 'thirty-mins obs', and again, had no idea what that meant. It meant that I had to be observed by one of the nurses every thirty minutes and, much to my horror, that was twenty-four hours a day! So, during the night, every thirty minutes, my room door would open and a nurse's head would pop in to 'observe' me. It was one of the many things in The Priory that would once in a while remind me that I was in an acute psychiatric hospital. Being moved from thirty-mins obs to one-hour obs, and then to two-hour obs was a real badge of honour amongst us 'inmates'. Sadly, but rightly, you were always under some sort of 'obs'.

After breakfast, we had our first group session. It was like being back at school but with a bunch of misfits from all walks of life. The great irony is that people with addictive behaviour issues are very often utterly self-obsessed. I certainly was, yet in The Priory everyone is the same. I came across gangsters, lawyers, prostitutes, doctors and even other professional sportspeople … but we were all the same. All having fallen to pieces, all with different stories, but all with a common thread of pain.

In our first session, I wasn't really expected to contribute but just listen. The therapist went around the room and asked people to share how they were feeling and where they were at with everything. The first person it went to was Lenny.

Almost as soon as he started to share his feelings, I started to cry. As he spoke, he also cried. This really hard man, who had seen the very worst of what the streets could do, was baring his heart and soul. He shared about how ashamed he was of the person he had become, and how he wanted to do better for his wife and children, whom he utterly adored. He talked about the loneliness he felt and how he knew there was a better person somewhere within him, but he just didn't know how get to that person. He felt trapped and didn't know where to start. I sobbed and sobbed as he spoke.

Lenny was the first person I had ever heard speak my language. He talked of the loneliness and shame that I had felt for years and years. I understood every single word and feeling he expressed. We were so different, yet so very much the same. There I was staring at a man that I would have claimed to have nothing in common with, yet he felt like a brother of mine. I was crying his pain and my pain, but I was also crying because I felt a little less alone in the world.

The most stunning part of Lenny's share was that he didn't care how vulnerable he looked. He had broken beyond caring what people thought of him. He talked about this though – he explained that in his world, showing weakness could have dire consequences, yet here in this hospital, with me and the others, he was letting go of that. I found it truly extraordinary.

The impact of Lenny's share lasted with me for days. I would go to my room and cry. I cried and cried for days. I felt like I had so much pain that needed to come out and tears were the best way of me doing this. The therapists always encouraged me to cry and never tried to interrupt me. I learnt that in group sessions it was best to let someone cry rather than place a hand or arm on them mid-cry. Although that was an act of support, it would also interrupt them from their tears.

Tears are healing, and I was often left to cry while knowing that people cared for me in the room.

***

A reflection of how deluded I was at the time was how long I initially wanted to stay at The Priory. I was told it was a twenty-eight-day programme and that it was strongly suggested I stay for that long. But I lived in this illusion that I was slightly better than most people – twenty-eight days, sure, but for me, it should only take seven days. I felt a seven-day stay would be enough for me. Looking back, it was utterly ridiculous. I was such a mess and yet I believed I could be 'fixed' in a quarter of the time that it would take other people. The great contradiction was that my self-esteem was shot and yet I still carried this huge ego with me.

This wasn't unusual for us patients, though. Denial was rife amongst us and discussions during mealtimes or coffee breaks would often centre on how things can't have been that bad. And this was amongst a group of people who had ruined marriages and families, been arrested, lost jobs, lost homes, were physically very poorly and were in their last of last chance saloons. There we were trying to convince everyone that actually we had everything under control! It was hilarious really, but only now can I see the absurdity of it all.

There were also people who were not willingly there. I had happily agreed to go but others are forced. Danny was one of these people. He was brought to The Priory about a week into my stay and when he was dropped off, he was smashed. He was a big tough man and was carried to his room by the nurses, his mum and his sister. It was hilarious to watch but there was also something so tragic about it. Once in his room, he was left to sleep it off. He awoke a bit later in the evening and had no idea where he was. He wandered into the main reception of the residential area and presumed he was in a hotel. The medical counter, where patients picked up their prescriptions, was also in the reception area. In his confusion, Danny thought the medical counter was a bar and sure enough, walked over to it and ordered himself a bottle of vodka! He was gently persuaded back to his room and to sleep!

However, when Danny woke up the next day fully sober it was clear he had no intention of staying. He didn't believe there was a problem and that his mum and sister had overreacted. He came to a handful of sessions, argued throughout all of them and eventually checked himself out. I've no idea where he is now or how things worked out. You can only pray that he is fine and has found peace in his life, but sometimes I do wonder about people like that.

I also watched as people changed very significantly in personality as they came off drugs or alcohol. It was my first experience of seeing how someone was one way when on, for example, heroine, and then a very different person once the drugs wore off. In the vast majority of cases this wasn't a pleasant thing to see. Andrea was in our group and she was lovely for the first couple of weeks – sweet, caring and really supportive of everyone there. By week three, the heroine had started to clear from her system and she became completely different. She would attack many of us verbally during group sessions and became more and more isolated. Underneath the heroine was a lot of anger within her and it was horrible to see. It is why therapists tell you that they can't treat the underlying issues until you stop whatever destructive behaviour you partake in.

Andrea was actually a big part of the reason that Lenny was thrown out of The Priory.

***

I thought Lenny was an amazing human being. He was thrust into a world of crime on the streets. He had no choice in that matter. While I was being pampered at Millfield School, he was just trying to survive in a tough part of Liverpool. He knew no other way.

He was fully aware that the way he earned a living wasn't something to be proud of and wanted something different for him and his family, but trying to step away from it was not as simple as leaving a job. He was part of a network that didn't cater for people trying to 'turn good'. Despite all of this he had a beautifully gentle heart. Not only did he look out for me from day one, but he also took himself off to the local shopping centre one night and bought everyone, including the nurses, presents.

However, the dark side of Lenny was that he had a lot of anger under the surface. He had seen a lot and carried a lot of emotional scars. Heroine had calmed him and coming off it meant him dealing with the person underneath. But he embraced that, and I loved him for it. He wanted to be the best version of himself he could be. Nonetheless, the anger was never far away.

Andrea had started to create a lot of problems within the group and Lenny wasn't reacting to it well. There was also another guy in the group called James, who bizarrely seemed to be winding up Andrea even more. She focused her anger and verbal barbs at me, Lenny and Johnny. Johnny was another friend of ours. A brilliant guy with more addictions than you could list.

I'm not really sure why Andrea disliked us so much, but I think our little group represented to her cocky men who thought we knew it all. Something within Andrea's psyche absolutely hated this and she was often coming after us. I found it quite funny and just a bit odd. Lenny didn't take it like that. He knew only one way when being attacked, and that was to attack back. It was his survival instinct from the streets but unfortunately it wasn't pretty.

During one group session, Andrea started to talk about how awful we were. Lenny had had enough. Not only did he let his mouth fly back at her, but he also threw a few chairs across the room. Chaos broke out and you were either in the Lenny part of the room or the Andrea part of the room, with the therapist trying to get calm back. I was firmly behind Lenny!

People started to leave the room and the therapist called for a break. We held Lenny back and Andrea walked out. We stayed in the room and tried talking it all through, but Lenny had seen his red mist. He felt that he and his friends were being attacked unfairly and there was only one answer for that. I begged Lenny to leave it but deep down I knew he wouldn't.

Andrea didn't come back to our group sessions that day but when we returned to the residential area, Lenny decided to finish off the discussion. The eye of his storm was now on James, who he felt had been acting as a snake in the whole situation. He pinned him against a wall and made it very clear what would happen to him if he ever crossed him again. Sadly, James reported Lenny to the duty manager and now a process was under way that Lenny wasn't going to win. The duty manager then called Lenny in and declared his behaviour unacceptable. Not one to take a backwards step, Lenny then threatened the duty manager. The end result was it was deemed that Lenny would have to leave The Priory immediately, even though he was due to stay for another three weeks.

I found it devastating. Lenny was also devasted and scared. He knew he wasn't ready for the outside world and desperately wanted to get better. You could see that there was a part of him that saw this as being life as per normal for him – he would always come off worse in the end. Lenny was trying to make a better life for himself and I suspected he had been trying to do this for a long while, but this was just another example in his eyes as to why this was impossible for him.

I helped him pack up his stuff in his room. His room was like the scene of a jail mate who had bribed the guards and had all the modern-day luxuries that were not allowed for normal inmates. As a result, it took some packing up. Lenny raged and cried throughout. I begged him to stick with his recovery path and I could tell there was a deep desire in him to do so. But at the same time, I could sense a fear in him. He didn't know how to survive in his environment without drugs. I guess we all felt like that in one way or another.

What Lenny did wasn't acceptable, but he knew no other way. He was defending himself and his friends and didn't know how to do this in a less aggressive manner. I went to see the duty manager myself and begged her to let Lenny stay. She was insistent that they couldn't have a situation where staff and patients felt unsafe. I understood but how were we to help someone like Lenny then? He was a good person who needed help.

Lenny was picked up by his wife and mum, and we said our goodbyes in the car park. I didn't know if I would see Lenny again. We all cried and hugged. I went back to my room and sobbed as I did on my first day. To start with, I couldn't understand why I was so affected by Lenny leaving. I realised in the end that it was because he was the first person who showed me that I wasn't alone in the world in how I felt. He showed me that compassion and empathy could work across people regardless of status or background. He was a flawed man, as we all are, but was trying to make a better person of himself. I found that inspiring.

Seeing Lenny go was really tough. There were a number of times that I wanted to do a runner from The Priory and this was definitely one.

Where did it start and finish for me to end up here?

Chapter 5

My planned seven-day stay in The Priory became fourteen days.

It wasn't like I was sold on the fact that I needed to stay for twenty-eight days, but I had started to recognise that I might need a little longer and I was definitely in a place that could help. As always, the greatest challenge for me was me. My ego, my feeling of self-importance and my deep sense that I was different to almost anyone else I ever met. All of this was preventing me from really understanding what was wrong with me and what I needed to change.

There was a great irony in this all. That feeling of being different was something I was very proud of. It is what I believed had made me survive and do well in the world. I remember being challenged by a girlfriend at university as to why I had trained until I vomited and then would party for four days. My answer: 'Because I am different to everyone else.'

This was a huge part of my persona within professional cricket. I would more often than not be playing against guys with more natural ability than me, but I held on to this belief that my 'difference' was my intensity and relentless attitude. And I wasn't making it up; that *was* my difference. I remember arriving at Lancashire CCC in 2005 and being in a changing room with world-class players. Freddie Flintoff had just won the Ashes with England and was a global superstar, and I had a conscious thought that the only way I would survive amongst these guys was to show them a level of intensity to cricket and life that they would respect. And the truth is that it worked.

But now my greatest strength was my greatest weakness. My inability to be able to accept that the help I needed was just like everyone else in there, was now my greatest threat.

To add to this, my belief at that time was also that if I sorted out all the problems I was dealing with then I would get better. I would drink less, be less anxious and generally happier. First and foremost, I needed to find some peace over Nia dying … then I had marriage difficulties, stress with work, stress with life, and hang-ups over boarding school. All of these things were making me feel the way I did and then causing me to behave the way I did.

That's what I thought, anyway.

I would list all these things to well-meaning friends and drinking buddies and, of course, it all sounded plausible. Especially the Nia card. How could a friend actually try to suggest anything other than that being a horrific moment in my life that would affect me for a lifetime?

There were some extraordinary therapists in The Priory at that time. Richard, Susie and Maggie were compassionate and highly skilled, and they saved my life. Their first challenge was to get me to see that my perspective (that I was different, and if you had my problems then you would behave the way I did) was actually killing me.

I thought that when I arrived at The Priory I had completely fallen apart – that thin piece of paper torn up into millions of little pieces. Little did I know that I was about to be broken down far more in order to rebuild me.

***

The aftermath of Lenny leaving was tough. The bond you build with your group peers is extraordinary. You pour your heart out to them and they know more about your life than anyone else in the world. You tell them every dark secret that lives within you and they don't judge you. They listen and relate, and you do the same with them. I cried many tears with my group peers and they did with me.

Once you are settled into some sort of routine at The Priory you are asked to write a life story, which you then read to the group. They emphasise to you that this needs to be the story of your difficulties. So, not a biography of your life but instead, a timeline of how you think your difficulties started and where they got to. They tell you again and again not to leave anything out.

You are given a couple of days to get this written and you will have heard a couple read out by other people before you do yours. Remembering everything was not a problem for me, it was the fact that I had to be completely honest with this group of strangers that was difficult. Truly honest. Not a version of the truth that you think will work. Unfortunately, the phrase 'Don't kid a kidder' is so true when people share their life stories to the group. Addicts are the world's leading experts in lying. They have lied most of their lives in order to survive, so they can smell bullshit a mile off! I had sat in life story sessions where group members openly told the person sharing that they weren't telling the whole truth, and the person was asked to try again with the life story. So I knew that I had to be entirely honest, and that was desperately hard.

I told them about all the big things, but I also told them about my hidden shames. I told them about the night I was left alone in the house with the twins when they were just over a year old. Precious, beautiful babies. All I had to do was be a vaguely responsible father and human being, and I couldn't do it. I remember Jude leaving the house that Saturday morning and I felt scared about what might happen. As much as I told myself that I wouldn't drink or do anything silly, there was a sense of inevitability deep in my gut. In the end I told myself that I could drink moderately, and all would be fine. I tried that and, of course, it failed. I woke up, having passed out on the kitchen floor, at 8.00 am. The twins were in their cots screaming for their lives and trying to climb out. They would have likely been awake for well over an hour. I had never told anyone about that. That's who I really was. The dark shame that lay within me. I wasn't a good person and I wasn't a good father.

I sobbed throughout reading my life story. I couldn't ever lift my eyes from the paper while I was reading, or after I had finished. I shook so hard that I had to put my paper on the table. Throughout it all, my peers cried with me and listened; they never interrupted or even made a sound. When I finished, the therapist, Maggie, said one thing to me: 'You're not a bad person, Luke, you're a poorly person.'

That's what no judgement feels like and I think it was the first time in my life when I truly felt that. These people didn't judge me at all for everything I told them. They empathised with me. My whole adult life had revolved around what everything looked like to the outside world. I was terrified of judgement. In fact, I was fast to judge others in order to avoid the focus being on me. Yet, here I was in a space where I had told people everything about me. I mean everything. And there was no judgement. It was extraordinarily powerful for me. I will never forget Maggie's words and the look in her eyes after I shared. She meant what she said. It was the first time in my life when I felt like there was a chance that I could tell people the truth and see what would come from it.

***

I came to realise that people were coming and going all the time from the hospital. Our group changed a great deal while I was there. Some people go on to another hospital, some don't want to be there, some complete the twenty-eight days, and some, like Lenny, get chucked out.

Johnny was someone who remained there throughout with me.

I had a lot in common with Johnny. We were about the same age with young families on the outside, with a marriage in serious difficulty. We also had huge egos! I am still friends with Johnny and love him to death. There are people you meet in rehab that you know you would have partied with on the outside and you laugh about it. Johnny was definitely one of those people. He was wild but had a really good heart. Like Lenny, he wanted to be a better man.

Johnny had a serious family history of addiction and suicide. There was this lineage within Johnny's life that he found so hard to break away from. He was desperate to break the cycle of the men before him, but you could sense he feared an inevitably of this pattern.

Johnny and I became great friends and he helped me massively. It wasn't like he had come anywhere close to overcoming his addictions, but he recognised what needed to be done before I did, and we would talk about it over thousands of cups of coffee. Johnny knew the problem lay within him. The problems he faced in life were of his own doing. He had his Nia card through his own family's tragedies but was telling me that the problem lay within him.

He wasn't quite in a place to deal with the problems within him but that change of perspective was really powerful to me. I remember repeating what he said to me again and again: 'Yeah but Luke, the problem lies within me.'

No excuses. He had made choices in life and the results were problems. He wasn't saying, like I told everyone, that if you had my problems you would behave and feel this way. He was taking responsibility.

We were always encouraged to spend lots of time with our group peers – mealtimes, coffee breaks, evenings etc. Of course, this is partly a measure for people to avoid isolating but it is also because there is something hugely powerful about one person sharing their truth with another person. I listened to Johnny because I saw him as similar to me. He understood me, and I understood him. When we talked and shared our thoughts and lives, we helped each other.

These sorts of influences really started to challenge my perception of what I was in The Priory for. I was holding on to a belief that I was there to rest, patch myself up, chat through a few of my problems, and then quickly get back into the world to show everyone how well I was. I was still living with this perception that the only thing that mattered was how things looked.

Even my perception of the truth was being challenged. The truth is the truth, but I started to realise that I considered it as a picture that I painted. These were subtle yet huge movements in my attitude to and perception of life.

***

During my second week at The Priory the fog had definitely started to clear in my mind, and I was becoming more aware of why I was there and where might be the problem, and therefore, where might lie the answer. I stress the word 'might' here. I wasn't convinced but it was certainly a consideration. I had also had a number of consecutive days of good sleep and food, and felt physically so much better.

On some weekdays, we had peer supporter sessions, which is where former patients would come back and run a session in which they would share their stories and help us with questions that we might have. No therapists were in the room.

These sessions were incredible. I found the peer supporters, or previous patients, utterly inspiring. They had walked the steps I had and looked so happy. They looked at peace with the world. They were happy in their stillness and shared a calmness that I found spellbinding. In the outside world, I remember I used to treat people with that level of self-assurance with deep suspicion. How were they so comfortable in their skin? What did they know that I didn't know? I would end up being as equally fascinated with them as I was suspicious of them.

They would tell us their stories, which would include suicide attempts, physical abuse, lost jobs, prison time, lost families, lost everything; they were just like us. And yet, there they stood in utter control of themselves. Completely comfortable with who they were and not at all bothered by what we might think of them. How could they be so disinterested in what people thought about them? I found it mind-blowing.

Anyway, I was still determined to leave after fourteen days. I had done another week and I felt miles better. I appreciated some of the concepts I had been taught and would follow them up, but it was time for me to get back out into the world. I certainly didn't want anyone to think that something was wrong with me.

On day thirteen I went to a peer supporter session where I met a lovely lady called Jane. She was Grade A in calmness and self-assurance. She told me about how she once locked herself in a bedroom while she drank and behaved like a wild animal. I actually started laughing because it sounded so absurd looking at this beautifully serene lady.

I started to regale about the problems I had, how I was ready to fix them and that it was time that I got back out there. I had a business to run, cricket to get back to – I was very important, didn't you know. She listened quietly, never showing a flicker of judgement or opinion, never interrupting or hurrying me. There was absolutely no edge to her.

Once I ran out of breath, she thanked me for sharing that, stared at me intensely but kindly, and simply said, 'Luke, just love yourself enough to stay here longer.'

At the time I had no idea why what she said had utterly gripped me. It was a pretty simple line after all. There was not much to the well-meaning sentence, but I was hooked to it for some reason. But I now understand. She was one of my peers and had been through the entire process and looked to be living the life I wanted to, and she had calmly listened to everything I had to say and had then said that I should stay in this hospital for longer. That meant she didn't think I was well enough to leave! It shattered the illusion in my head that I was ready to go home. It was actually a hammer blow to my ego. There was no way I could attack her opinion as she epitomised what I wanted in life. I had to take it on board.

The second part was that she asked me to love myself enough to stay. That meant I didn't love myself enough. But in my head, I did – I was a leader, a captain, a business owner; I was different! So that meant she was referring to loving something else within me. She was asking me to tap into myself. My soul. Forget about what people thought, just start loving the person I was deep down enough to try to rebuild my life.

It might all sound simple, but it was earth-shattering for me.

When the session finished, I thanked Jane and walked back to the residential area in the pouring rain. I was alone, and I sobbed my heart out. I knew what the problem was. I probably had all along but, for the first time, I was saying it openly.

The problem was ME.

I called my mum and dad on the way back as I cried and said, 'I really need to stay longer; I need to do the full twenty-eight days.'

I finally realised that I was in exactly the right place and I was here to start fixing me. This was an inside job. Forget everyone else; this was about me and what lay within my soul and attitude to life. There was another sense of relief about this decision but also a great deal of fear.

I had no idea what lay ahead.

If I wasn't to be the person I thought I was, then who was I?

Chapter 6

My childhood was loving and colourful, and took me all over the world. Like with anyone, it moulded my thoughts and beliefs of the world. It was always going to play a part in my progress at The Priory.

***

My father, David, worked for an oil company throughout his working life, which meant we travelled the world, living in countries where gas and oil reserves existed. My earliest memories as a boy were living in Oman, in the Middle East. My dad worked there for eleven years and I actually travelled out there with my mum when I was six weeks old. However, I guess my earliest memories would have been from when I was about 4 years old.

Oman was a really friendly, peaceful and crime-free country. We grew up in a safe and carefree atmosphere. I remember exploring the 'wadi', which is the Arabic word for a valley, near our house with my brother, Noel, who is five years older than me. We would venture off and explore in and around the rocks. I remember the heat, the smell and texture of the land. It was rough and full of mystery. I loved it. My brother is my hero and that feeling of us sharing that adventure and warmth on our backs was wonderful. We were always keeping an eye out for scorpions and snakes, but that early closeness to nature was amazing. Incidentally, my brother once got bitten on the bum by a scorpion, which we managed to capture and get frozen into a glass case. The scorpion glass case sat proudly in our house for many years. Not a terribly interesting story, but I'm enjoying embarrassing my brother!

I also remember swimming in Oman. I recall the lovely feeling of the heat and the water on my skin as we swam in the pool. To this day, I still feel a huge resonance with the water, nature and warmth of the sun.

Prior to Oman, my parents had lived in Nigeria, where they were temporarily evacuated during the civil war. For my mum, Molly, this was a particularly huge shock venturing into the big wide world. She comes from a fairly traditional Irish Catholic family and married young. Suddenly they were living in Africa and experiencing the realities of a bloody civil war. In the past I have taken for granted the number of experiences my parents have shared around the world. They were adults, but it was also moulding their perspective on the world and parenthood. As a family in the 1980s, we were living a wonderful but unusual life compared to others.

We stayed in Oman until I was 5 years old and then moved to Peru and lived the capital, Lima. This is where my most profound early childhood memories are from. I absolutely loved Peru and remember so much about it.

If Oman was carefree and peaceful, then Peru was very different. The Falklands conflict broke out while we were mid-air on our way there. The atmosphere was noisy, hostile and a bit frightening at times, but nonetheless, we settled in quickly and lived a really good expat life. The two houses we lived in during our time there were big, and we had all the trappings of foreigners working and earning well in the country. We would go to the county club at the weekend and had a live-in housekeeper called Gladys. Granted, it wasn't quite living the authentic Peruvian life, but it was still a huge cultural experience for us all.

As with Oman, there was the heat and the ruggedness of playing outside most of the time. There were so many new experiences for me in Peru. For starters, it was the first time that I began to use a different language – Spanish. I went to a school, Markham College, that mixed English and Spanish equally, and I talked to most of my friends in Spanish. In many ways, Spanish became my first language. I remember cringing while listening to my parents speak Spanish; they sounded so 'foreign'. I was often used as the translator with the gardener or someone similar who spoke no English. To this day, I love Spanish and, as strange as it might sound, it feels very comforting for me to hear and speak the language.

My Spanish was greatly improved by Gladys. By this time, my brother had gone to boarding school in England at Wells Cathedral School, so I hung out with Gladys a lot. She had very dark skin and big Afro hair. She was a strict Catholic, gentle and fun. I only ever spoke Spanish to her and I adored her. Gladys looked different to us, spoke differently, lived a different sort of life, and was amazing. It was such an important learning experience for me at that age, giving me appreciation that the world is full of different sorts of people and to respect people for that difference.

We had a giant tortoise called Solomon who would walk across the garden with me on his back. He'd never eat his lettuce until you had moved out of sight. We had a couple of dogs – Sammy, who, heartbreakingly, ran away, and Lobo, a wild Doberman. We inherited Lobo with the second house we lived in. She had had a tough life up till then. She wasn't calm, and my dad definitely couldn't go near her without risking losing a limb, but she liked me, I think because I was small and didn't intimidate her. Unfortunately, the gardener let her run loose one day and she bit someone running past the house, so she had to be taken away. I remember crying my eyes out when she was picked up. She was terrifying and would absolutely guarantee that no one would come near the front door who wasn't welcome, but she was sweet to me.

Crime was always a concern in Lima. I remember the busy, dirty roads, where people would approach the cars at traffic lights to sell you newspapers or wash your windscreens. It was a huge no–no to ever leave your arm resting on full show with the window open. Any sort of watch would be taken off your wrist in a less than gentle fashion. Machetes to the wrist were sadly not unknown. If you visited the markets, then money would need to be hidden in your underwear and no jewellery could be visible.

Peru was also where I first started to swim seriously. I joined a swimming club and started to get really good at it. It became a huge part of mine and my parents' social life. It was when I noticed how much of a 'gringo' I was in Peru. That's the Spanish nickname for someone with blond hair and fair skin – generally foreigners! My bright blond hair made me stand out a mile when swimming against my darker Peruvian counterparts. There wasn't a cricket ball in sight at this time, but I was becoming a very promising swimmer.

We would travel all over Lima for swimming competitions and I fell in love. I was immediately hooked on the nature of competition. As my mum will testify, I was a pretty full-on child at times, so competition was perfect for me to direct my energy towards. I loved the anticipation of the race. Turning up to the venue, checking everything out, wondering who your competition was and having that slight fear of not knowing what would happen. By the way, I was definitely not turning up to just take part! I had a natural intensity about winning from 6 or 7 years old.

Even on race days, there was an allure about the water for me. As I waited for the starter's gun while crouched on the block at the start of the race, I would feel this tingling sensation across my skin. There was momentary dead silence and I would hear the water lapping in the pool. I would feel the air on my skin and just wanted that sensation of diving into the water. The draw to the water and, importantly, to the race was huge for me. It felt so natural.

And I would win a lot. I was really good and had a ferocious appetite to win every race. I ended up with lots of junior trophies and medals, and loved the acknowledgement of winning … possibly too much at times. If, God forbid, I didn't win, then I most definitely was not a gracious loser! Losing was not part of the calculus for me. I felt at home in the water and even more so while racing.

Peru was full of so many happy experiences, including a trip to Machu Pichu with the whole family, but it was also the first time that I was without my brother for long periods. Noel was now at boarding school in England and would come to see us, or vice versa, in the school holidays. I have always worshipped my brother and he was very protective of me. I think that five-year age gap was a blessing for me and a curse for him at times. Whichever key stage my brother got to,

I was always that annoying younger brother – 8 years old to his 13; 13 to his 18; 16 to his 21!

During one of the school holidays, my brother had come back to Peru and came to pick me up from school with my mum. I was so happy to see him. It coincided with a time at school when we had discovered these plant seeds, which if you scraped on the ground and then touched someone's skin would sting to high hell. I had been chased around all day by various school bullies and was obviously not coping with it that well. When my brother turned up, he noticed that I was being chased and promptly began chasing down the bullies to protect me. What an absolute god he was to me! My hero, my older brother, a total legend in my eyes.

But this was a time when I began getting used to having lots of time apart from Noel. I was surrounded by love and attention, particularly from my mum, but the majority of those early memories in Peru were without Noel. I recognise now that these were some important dynamics happening in my early life. I was getting used to being without a significant person, and having to learn how to get on without their protection, and at the same time was receiving unfettered attention from my parents, particularly my mum.

Peru was just one big adventure and I loved every minute of it. When the time came for my parents to tell me that we were leaving, I was really upset. It felt like so many foundations had been established in my life in Peru and now it all had to change. Moving from place to place was the life we led with my dad's job and it came with some amazing benefits. But the moving was a tough part of it. Friendships that were formed were realistically over, and we had to start all over again in a new country. There was an excitement about moving, but Peru had meant so much to me.

***

Our next stop was The Hague in Holland. I was now 8 years old and Noel was still at boarding school in England. Holland was such a different experience to much of what my life had been up till then. It was my first time living in Europe. To begin with, most people spoke English! In fact, it was much more like England, where we would regularly visit in school holidays. I went to the British School in The Hague and we lived in an apartment right up against the beachfront in a place called Scheveningen.

I found Holland such an interesting country; it had so much colour and personality. There was different food but also the same. For example, most people love pancakes but in Holland they actually have restaurants that only serve pancakes. *Pannenkoekenhuis* or Pancake House – genius! It was also the first place that I could openly have chocolate at breakfast, in the form of chocolate sprinkles. I have always loved cheese but in Holland, we were going to another level. As for mayonnaise on chips, the Dutch made this an art form.

The tulip fields, the windmills, the clogs, the canals, the history … there was just so much to absorb and love in Holland. It was worlds apart from Peru but, as a child, you quickly adapt and move on.

I got straight into the swimming culture in Holland by joining a club and doing lots of racing, and my parents joined a squash club at Klein Zwitserland. We all settled in really quickly. I started to make new friends and life was fun. I had a Danish friend called Peter, who loved football and started to tell me all about it. We would go down to the beachfront and practise penalties against each other for hours and hours. My dad has always had a unique whistle for my brother and me, and he could lean out of our balcony and whistle down the beachfront and I knew it meant time to come home. Many an early evening would involve a marathon penalty shootout followed by one of my dad's whistles.

My swimming really took off in Holland. The swimming club I joined was very competitive and I guess I was seen as one of the rising stars. I was winning more and more, and eventually the opportunity for me to swim in the National Championships came about. Breaststroke was my style at that time and I basically believed I was unbeatable! I have no doubt that I would have been very annoying to other people. I lived and breathed winning. I was hooked on the feeling it gave me. Of course, I loved the water, and winning a race in it was an irresistible combination for me.

I went to the National Championships with my mum and dad and had no other expectation than that I would win. The race was in a 50 metre pool rather than a 25 metre pool in which I normally swam. The 50 metre pool looked a mile long but I genuinely didn't think there would be any other result than me winning. Even at 7 or 8 years old, I really did have a belief that I was a bit different to everyone else. If I'm totally honest, I thought I was a bit better than everyone else.

I remember the race. I remember being in the highest graded lane as the fastest qualifier. I remember pushing hard at the start and being at the front. I also remember not being out in the lead as per normal. I remember people being close and me fighting through the water. I remember feeling a struggle for the rhythm and the lead.

I remember finishing forth.

Fourth.

My poor parents. They must have watched on so proudly and then known that fourth was never going to cut it with me, and they would be dealing with the aftermath. There was absolutely no gracious loser in me. There were tears, tantrums, the full works. I'm actually cringing as I write this.

I can still remember the photo of the podium and me on the end of it in fourth place. The lad who won had the broadest smile and looked a bit like the cute kid from the film *Jerry Maguire*. He was so happy, and I would have happily pushed him off the podium. I was a bloody nightmare!

I would love to say that my attitude towards not winning changed from that experience, but it definitely didn't. I expected full adulation from winning every time I competed. I remember one Christmas organising a family snooker tournament. My mum was unfortunately the weakest player and someone with an ounce of grace would probably take it easy on her. Oh no. The tournament was organised, by me, so that the overall winner would have the highest aggregate number of points from all three of their matches. In my mind this meant I needed to rack the points up against my mum. No mercy was shown; she was the weak link and I completely wiped her out! I duly won the tournament.

I had also begun to play squash in Holland, mainly against my dad and brother. My dad was obviously miles better and would take it easy on both of us. My brother and I were reasonably close, but he was a bit better. I would literally break myself trying to win, particularly against my brother. My T-shirt would be completely drenched in sweat and I'd be gasping for air. If I lost, which I did a fair bit, the wrestle that would ensue with my T-shirt would have been comical to watch. I would have such a tantrum that my T-shirt was the only thing I could vent against. A damp T-shirt stuck to your skin makes a very tough opponent during a pathetic tantrum. I still remember my dad's words one day: 'It's not your T-shirt's fault!'

I went through a period when I couldn't beat my brother at Connect Four. I was certain he was cheating (I am still suspicious). It drove me wild! I would play him again and again, obsessed with winning. Same result every time, but I wouldn't give up.

The single-mindedness within me was so strong at an early age. In Holland, it really came to life. I was good at sport and that combined with my obsession with winning meant I was always going to be a competitor of some sort.

Living in Holland was another wonderful experience for me, but it also signalled the time for a big change in my life … boarding school.

***

My parents are really good people. My dad is wise, calm and very kind. My mum is passionate, fiercely loyal and hugely compassionate. The bond with my mum at that age was strong. Mo, as I called her, was the centre of my world. I had had her full attention for much of my life and she always gave me the belief and spirit to be the competitor I was. My mum absolutely believed in me.

They were faced with a really tough choice. My dad had a fantastic job that provided for the family really well, but it also meant a lot of travel. They knew that Holland would come to an end soon and, in the same way that it was for my brother, they felt they couldn't risk my schooling being so broken up in different parts of the world. I also had little knowledge of the UK and not much of a relationship with my extended family because of where we had lived until then. I know my mum worried about how the course of my life would be affected if anything happened to her and dad. I was also showing strong signs of being a very good sportsman, particularly a swimmer.

When the opportunity came about for me to go to Millfield School – or Edgarley Hall, as the prep school was called then – it seemed an obvious choice in many ways. Millfield had a phenomenal sporting history and were willing to offer me a swimming scholarship. My brother was also still at boarding school in Wells, which wasn't a million miles from Millfield.

In the end the decision for me to go to Millfield as a boarder seemed a natural one. I now understand why my parents made that choice. It was really difficult for them and they made the best possible call in their eyes. I love and respect them for that, but there is no doubt it had a big impact on me. I can vividly remember being dropped off at my new boarding house, The Mews, and trying to settle in with other 9-year-olds I had never met. It was a bright sunny day, and everything seemed absolutely terrifying. All the children and parents were arriving with trunks full of clothes and there was that bristle of energy around the boarding house. I just didn't want to say goodbye to my parents. I can't imagine the turmoil it would have put them through. It would have absolutely killed my mum.

For me, it was heartbreaking. I loved my dad but being separated from my mum was absolutely horrific. As I write these words, tears are streaming down my face. I remember the feeling and it was so hard. I didn't want to say goodbye to Mo; she was everything to me. Dorm 9 was my new home with four other boys, one of whom was older. James was 12 but seemed like he was 25. We were all terrified, but we just had to get on with it.

During the first week you were only allowed one ten-minute call home. I couldn't bear it. When the day came for our call, we all queued up one by one outside the phone and took our turn. Hearing my mum's voice was as heartwarming as it was heartbreaking. I literally begged her over and over again to pick me up. Again, I can't imagine what that was doing to her. She calmly explained that she couldn't do that and things would get better, and that I would see them soon. It was just so much for me to take at that age. Mo used to write to me all the time and I loved getting an envelope with her handwriting on it. She would always sign it off 'Mo' and I would keep the cards next to my bed all the time.

Once you got to the second weekend of boarding, you were allowed to go on exeat. This meant you could go away from the school for the weekend. This was a Saturday lunchtime pick-up and a Sunday night return. My mum came back to England to pick me up and I will never forget that feeling. I remember walking into the school car park after lessons (we had lessons on Saturday mornings) had finished, frantically looking for my mum. I couldn't find her and I was panicking. I was frantic.

And then I saw her and have never felt a feeling like it. We hugged and kissed and cried and cried. I was so happy to see her.

It was wonderful to go home with my mum that weekend to talk, cuddle and eat her food. I had missed her horrendously. But waking up on Sunday morning meant going back to school at the end of that day. It was a mini repeat of the first time I was dropped off. That separation from my mum was so hard for me to take.

Just like it was when my brother went away, this was the start of me getting used to coping without a significant person in my life to protect me. In fact, with my mum, it was the most significant person in my life by a country mile. Mo was the centre of my universe.

This, however, was the start of a ten-year adventure.

And that adventure was Millfield School.

Chapter 7

T wo things I know for sure about Millfield School:

I have never been in an environment like it since leaving.

And I would never have become a professional cricketer without going there.

***

Millfield School is a truly extraordinary institution. I still meet with and speak to old schoolmates in the big wide world, and there is not one of us who doesn't reflect back on Millfield without a sense of wonderment about our time there.

But this isn't all good.

It is a completely unique school that offers incredible opportunities and instils an amazing attitude towards competition, but with boarding, that can bring with it challenges. I am enormously grateful for what Millfield offered me but there is no doubt that my ten years there left some scars that needed dealing with during my time in The Priory.

***

My life at Millfield started at the prep school Edgarley Hall, and with my scholarship, I quickly joined the elite swimming programme. We would train five days a week, always early in the morning and always at the senior school. That meant a 5.30 am rise and then a cold walk in the dark to the minibus. It was horrible. In the heart of winter, there was very little to make you want to do that. Despite the money at the school, the pool at the senior school at that time was not the incredible facility you see now. It was a very tired 33.3 metre pool with a hard plastic dome covering. Hardly inviting! To make matters worse, the changing rooms were outside the pool so you had to walk across in the cold in your swimming trunks. Millfield was exceptional at producing elite swimmers and this was by no means a pampered programme.

When I refer to the programme being elite, I'm not necessarily referencing the actual coaching or the training, which incidentally was very good. It was the mentality. And that mentality was all over Millfield. It was the epitome of a winning mentality. We wore Millfield Swimming T-shirts when we went to competitions and they simply said, 'We Swim Fast'. And that was it – we swam fast, we were better than you and we made no apology for it. That attitude irritated lots of other people but we didn't care. The whole ethos was around winning and that we were better than everyone else. There was no room for any other attitude.

My school hockey coach, Tim Wilbur, whom I loved, once said to me, 'We're always 1–0 up before we get on the field.' I asked him why and his answer was, 'Because we are Millfield.' That elite mentality to everything was incredibly powerful. Millfield helped me hugely to become a professional cricketer and the vast majority of this came from the mentality it instilled in me. I went into the school as a swimmer and left as a cricketer, but the mentality was consistent throughout. It wasn't about taking part; it was about winning.

I was perfect for Millfield: a highly competitive young boy who had natural sporting ability. I had entered an environment that would bring out the best in me in sporting terms. It was boosting my confidence and encouraging me not to be apologetic about being ferociously competitive.

There was often talk amongst the swimming squad that there were three S's when you were a swimmer – Swimming, Schoolwork and Social life. Most of the time, you would only be able to have two out of three, and swimming was non-negotiable, so one of the others would have to suffer. This wasn't discouraged by anyone; it was the mentality we all bought into and understood. It was the way it was and why it was the perfect preparation for professional sport. The sport came first and everything else came after.

While in The Priory, I would learn that my attachment to being successful brought out both the best and the worst in me. I was defined by being successful or, at least, appearing successful. I would also learn that it would give me the affirmation I craved. All of this would come back to bite me eventually, but it was also going to make me the best possible sportsperson I could be.

***

Boarding is like being thrown in at the deep end.

We had amazing matrons, sort of 'mums' away from our mums, and lots of other pastoral care, but the very nature of boarding is tough at a young age. What quickly develops is that your peers – initially your dorm mates – become hugely important. You are all in it together and so the bond that builds between you is extraordinary. Paul Gillmon was one of my first dorm mates and we are still very close friends to this day. You cry together, sleep together, laugh together and find out so much about yourselves together. Your peers are the people you rely on because your parents are not there. This isn't a slight on Millfield's boarding; it is actually the very nature of boarding, especially from an early age.

Those first two weeks at Edgarley Hall were emotionally so hard, and the first month felt like a year long. Being away from my parents was really tough but I did settle at some point, although I can't remember exactly when. There was so much to do at the school that you couldn't help but get on with things.

I had travelled a lot throughout my life up till then, but this was a whole new world. There was so much to take in. Everything was big and bold – the facilities, the pupils and the opportunities. It felt massive – and I was only at the prep school!

I was obviously straight into the swimming at the school, but I also was introduced to all the other sports, many of which I had hardly played. We definitely hadn't played cricket or rugby in Peru. I loved it all and wanted to try everything. It never mattered what sport it was, there was always this distinct Millfield mentality to it. It was intoxicating. There was always an expectation that we would win and the intensity around the sporting teams was very strong. I thrived in that environment.

At the start of the summer term, all the boys who wanted to play cricket were brought together to talk about the Under 9s Edgarley Hall cricket team. The teacher in charge said, 'So, who would like to be the wicketkeeper?'

I had no idea what he was talking about and looking around the group, nor did anyone else. But no one put up their hand.

'Come on, every team needs a wicketkeeper. Who's going to do it?'

No one budged. Suddenly I realised that if every team needed a wicketkeeper and no one wanted to do it, then this was my guarantee into the team. I had no real idea about what it involved but I was sure as hell going to get myself in the team.

My hand shot up and sure enough, I became Edgarley Hall's Under 9s wicketkeeper. Little did I know then that this would become my job for the best part of twenty years.

As I made my way through the prep school, I certainly became more and more used to boarding. I adjusted to being away from my parents. As an example, we used to have to write a letter home on Saturdays in order to get our 'tuck bag'. A tuck bag was a paper bag of sweets that you had already ordered and would be allowed to eat on Saturday night in front of a movie. But in order to get your bag you had to write a letter to your mum and dad and present it to your house master. In the early days, my letters would be full of emotion and fairly long, but as time went on, they got shorter and shorter as all I wanted was my tuck bag as soon as possible! It was just a reflection that I was happy and becoming more independent from my parents.

Looking back, this independence was both good and bad. You learn to deal with challenges by yourself or with the help of your peers, simply because your mum and dad are not there to hold your hand through it. You become very resourceful and there is a great strength in this. But you definitely develop a pattern of not reaching out for help from your parents when you may do otherwise. It's a survival thing.

I would wet the bed fairly regularly in my first year of boarding and would desperately try to hide it from everyone. I would end up trying to get my bed sheets sorted quietly by myself. I never wanted to make a fuss about it by telling my mum and would just deal with it myself. This pattern of behaviour carried me through to when I was at university. I crashed a girl's car on campus while messing around one night when I was drunk. I didn't have the money to repair the damage, but I definitely didn't go to my parents for help. I leaned on my peers and found a way to resolve it myself.

There was actually so much that was positive about this resourcefulness and independence, but later in life it would mean that when I most needed help from people beyond myself and my peers, I wouldn't reach out as I should have done. I thought I could fix everything.

***

I really enjoyed my time at Edgarley Hall. I felt like I had progressed in so many ways. I had even started to meet girls! Weirdly, my swimming didn't flourish to the same extent. I think there were just so many distractions and other opportunities at the school that I didn't maintain the appetite for it that was needed. By the time I was leaving Edgarley Hall to go to the senior school, cricket was definitely the leading sport in my world.

So, at the age of 12, I moved on to the senior school, Millfield. If I thought Edgarley Hall was big and bold, I was hardly ready for what was coming next. Millfield was like a sensory overload on steroids. Everything was ridiculously massive.

The facilities were mind-blowing; the sixth-formers seemed like full-blown men and women. Everyone looked so cool – it was fucking terrifying! Edgarley Hall had a cuteness to it but Millfield just felt bold and brash.

The school was more of an American-style university campus – huge grounds with the flow of pupils controlled by a tannoy system. Everything looked incredible. Fellow pupils included children of celebrities and foreign princes and princesses. It was not unknown for a bodyguard to sit in a lesson with you keeping an eye on one of your classmates. As well as all of this, there were sportsmen and women who were already competing on a world level. And that Millfield mentality was still there, but times a billion!

The main rugby/football pitch was right in the middle of the school and we would all go to watch the first team play. The intensity around these matches and the admiration for the players was on another level. In our eyes they were like gods. It made you want to be out there winning and being loved for it. Being an elite sportsperson at Millfield felt like the greatest affirmation you could get. The same applied to all sports. There was a deep sense of history and culture. The whole school had an aura that was both terrifying and inspiring at the same time.

Never had my peers been so important to me, especially the ones that had come up from the prep school with me. We were like lemmings, absolutely terrified of being eaten by one of the Tyrannosaurus Rex sixth-formers. Everyone looked so confident and cool. And the girls were beautiful. In fact, I had never seen so many beautiful girls in one place.

Despite all my competitiveness on the sporting field, I was a really nervous teenager. At Millfield, appearance mattered greatly. I know that at all schools there is a pressure amongst pupils to look cool, but at Millfield it was intense. The school was awash with money and there wasn't a set school uniform, so it wasn't uncommon for boys to be wearing Armani or Hugo Boss suits, and many of the girls felt they couldn't wear the same outfit more than once. Some pupils would walk around with big sums of cash, and at times, it felt like it was an even contest between the obsession to look good and the desire to achieve sporting greatness.

I found the whole thing really daunting, but I did well, particularly with my cricket. Having been close to the England Under 14s team,

I became captain of England Under 15s. Of course, I received recognition about this at school but the competition for sporting achievement was fierce. Sixth-formers were leaving the school to go straight into professional sport. World-level competitions were in reach for the swimmers. It really was the elite of the elite.

Millfield wasn't a standard institution, but it wasn't designed to be. It was a school that created an environment in which to produce the best, and it could certainly do that. My hockey coach, Tim Wilbur, had a huge influence on me at the school. He also taught me history, which I loved, so I guess he had an added advantage. I had flirted towards challenging for the England Under 14s/Under 15s hockey squad, but I was pretty ordinary compared to most at that level and mainly hung in there through sheer determination. Mr Wilbur, or 'Wilbs', as we called him, became a father figure for me at Millfield in many ways. He believed in me, more for my mentality than for my ability. He encouraged me to be a leader with my attitude and determination. I felt he trusted me. He genuinely had a profound influence on me.

Wilbs was the first coach that I vomited for after a fitness test, having pushed myself to that extreme. He didn't try to slow me down but admired me for it. I was to go on and vomit after many fitness sessions throughout my professional sporting career. He encouraged that intensity in me and didn't make me feel odd for it. On the other hand, if I stepped over the line behaviourally, he was fast to come down on me. I had this pathetically petulant habit of throwing my hockey stick on the ground if something didn't go my way. He would be quick to haul me off the field if I behaved like that and I was told in no uncertain terms that it was unacceptable. I also went a bit astray when I was 16–17 years old. Girls had become an obvious distraction and I lost my focus for cricket, and all sport, for that matter. Wilbs was very fast to pull me in and get me back in line.

During my final year at Millfield, our hockey first team won the Indoor and Outdoor Under 18s National Championships. To this day, they are two of my proudest achievements. The school had never done that double up till then. I played left wing. Yes, left wing! I was hardly controlling the game in the middle of the field. Actually, left wing was the position no one else wanted to play. But it became mine, and Wilbs encouraged me to bring a level of energy to it that would completely disrupt the opposition. At the time, most attacks in hockey came from the right-hand side, so as a left winger, you were actually the first line of defence. I just threw myself at it. Wilbs wrote in my final school report that if he had eleven Luke Suttons he would win the National Championships every year. I had never felt prouder reading those words.

The greatest lesson that Wilbs taught me is that you can overcome limited ability through sheer determination, attitude and presence. He didn't make me feel like a bit-part player because I wasn't as talented as others, he made me feel like a leader with the attributes I had. The lessons I learnt from him carried me through my cricket career. At the moment I arrived at Lancashire CCC, surrounded by world-class players, my mind went to those crucial lessons I had learnt at Millfield in order to survive and thrive in that environment.

***

As I was coming to the end of my time at Millfield, I had started having more and more involvement with the local professional cricket club, Somerset CCC. I played my first second team game for them at 16 years old and was showing the possible pedigree to become a full-time professional, but it definitely wasn't guaranteed at this stage. I was still prone to being distracted by girls and nights out. Even then there were some warning signs that I couldn't necessarily control things when I started drinking. I went off to Durham University and was coached under the brilliant Graeme 'Foxy' Fowler. It was more of the same at Durham – I worked hard and played even harder. University was perfect for my drinking habits. My habit of playing just as hard on and off the field was fully established by now. It featured me missing my train to Shropshire for an England Under 18s training camp because I had been so drunk the night before and taking a taxi from Durham instead! There were numerous other semi-amusing/semi-disastrous episodes.

Ultimately, I was very lucky that Dermot Reeve took a punt on me and offered me my first professional contract with Somerset CCC in my first year out of Millfield. All the grounding I had at Millfield prepared me perfectly for surviving in professional sport. Once that door was opened for me, I didn't look back.

I now understand the impact that boarding at Millfield had on me. Some of it was gloriously amazing, and some of it came back to haunt me when my life began to unravel.

The mentality that was instilled in me gave me a fierce determination to survive in professional sport. I knew I wasn't as talented as many others, but it was in my blood to fight for a win. That was all that was important and everything else came second place.

I was consumed by success and absolutely defined myself by it. The affirmation I received from success is what I believed was real. As long as people admired me for my achievements then all was good in the world and I was a good enough person. There was sadly little depth beyond that.

Appearance mattered to me. It was part of my need to be defined by success. I was obsessed by what people thought about me. If they thought I was cool and a good person, then so did I! My need for affirmation was extraordinary and so I was equally obsessed with controlling what people thought of me.

I had learnt to survive on my own. It gave me great strength in difficult circumstances, but it also meant I believed I could handle and control everything. I didn't need help. Even when life was unravelling at an alarming rate, I still held on to the belief that I didn't need to reach out for help. I was the master of my own ceremonies. My addiction to control was just as damaging as anything else.

There was truly so much I was going to discover about myself during my final two weeks at The Priory.

Chapter 8

Richard was the lead therapist throughout my time at The Priory. He was abrasive at times. He was strong and happy to challenge anyone in a debate. He took no shit. And taking into consideration the amount of full-time bullshitters who walked through their doors, it was some effort. During my time there, Richard was admired and loathed in equal measures by the patients. He was also a recovering addict himself.

Richard was amazing for me and I'm very grateful for the time he gave me. Throughout my entire four weeks at The Priory, I always had this nagging feeling in the back of my head that maybe I was wasting everyone's time; maybe I wasn't that bad and really just needed a couple of good sleeps to crack on. The level of identification I would get from fellow patients during sessions would counteract that denial in me, but so did the time Richard gave to me. I felt like he understood me and knew I needed help to find a different way to lead my life.

During my first week we had one particularly lively group session. As you can imagine, lively sessions were never far away bearing in mind the room was full of maniacs detoxifying at different levels. This session was being led by an amazing therapist called Susie, but Richard walked in and interrupted it. Our group at this time was full of testosterone-driven men, including me, who Richard showed not the slightest inclination of being intimidated by.

'OK you lot, I think we need to have a really good chat about why you're all here and what you want to get out of your time in The Priory.'

This was at the time that Danny had been involuntarily dropped off at the hospital and was now arguing why he shouldn't be there. I was set on leaving at the end of the week, Lenny was struggling with the overall authority at the place, Phil thought the whole thing was a big con and Johnny was still waiting to be properly diagnosed so was up and down like a yoyo. Richard's challenging opening statement went down like a lead balloon.

'What do you mean?' one of us said.

'Well, you all think you know better than me and the other therapists, so you might as well fucking leave now.'

It was like a match to dynamite. It all kicked off.

Danny immediately demanded to leave. Phil started debating whether The Priory was worth the money. Lenny hated the affront and started shouting back. And, obviously, embarrassingly, I started crying.

The session fell apart. Danny walked out and discharged himself. But for the rest of us, Richard had basically called our bluff. If we thought we knew better and could cope in the outside world then we were free to leave. It was actually a terrifying position to be in. Deep down we knew that we were fucked and didn't know better, but it was just so ingrained in us to lead with our egos and believe we could control everything. Richard had clearly decided that it was time to risk losing people to change the dynamic in the group and save a few others. He just dropped a bomb in the group.

This moment is actually what convinced me to stay for another week. Richard suddenly made it very real to me that I was welcome to go back out into the world and try to survive on my own. I knew I couldn't.

I didn't just cry; I actually lost it for a bit. There was a little kitchen near the rooms where sessions took place and I took myself in there and sobbed my heart out. I gripped the sink and cried uncontrollably. I was so torn between who I thought I was and the notion that I might need to take a leap of faith and try something different. It was absolutely like standing on the edge of the cliff and deciding whether to jump. Not jumping would mean I would remain in the shit, but jumping meant not knowing where I would land. Part of my brain wanted to stick with the shit I knew, and the other part of my brain knew that I had to find a different way.

Richard walked into the kitchen.

'You OK, Luke? Shall we sit out in the sun in the garden?'

Now The Priory might not have had Jacuzzis, but it had damn nice gardens! We sat out on two chairs and Richard rolled up one of his customary cigarettes. It was a fresh but beautiful day. We talked about what had just happened in the group and I started to try to convince Richard why I was ready to leave after seven days. He basically ignored my rabbling and simply asked me, 'What makes you happy, Luke?'

A simple question but, by God, a difficult one to answer. I immediately had that moment of trying to think of things that I should say that would sound good. But I was facing Richard, who could see through bullshit before it came out of your mouth, so I just said the most natural thing that popped into my head: 'Being successful'.

There was a long pause as we looked at each other and then Richard said, 'Remember that answer, Luke. One day you will look back on this and understand what it is all about.'

At the time, I didn't have a clue what he meant but that simple answer perfectly illustrated where I was at. Some people might say spending time with their children, spending time with their wife, walking their dogs, eating a beautiful meal, watching football, painting, singing, dancing … basically anything other than 'being successful'!

That's how I defined myself. That's what I believed made people like me. If I was being successful, then all was good in the world.

'Luke, have you ever heard of the phrase "having a hole in your soul"?'

I didn't have a clue what Richard was talking about. He explained to me that finding a new way to live was a journey to truly finding myself. A journey to find out who I was deep in my soul. 'Being successful' was an example of me looking out for affirmation, rather than being comfortable with who I was as a person. I needed people to tell me that I was a good person so that I could then believe it. I didn't actually know who I was. I thought all the answers to my problems were outside of me, but they weren't; they were inside of me. That's why I was so sensitive about what people thought of me. It was the very essence of how I got my own self-worth. It was why I could fit into any crowd, because I wanted to fit into every crowd, and I had to fit into every crowd so that people liked me. I could put a mask on to fit whatever occasion was needed because it was all about appearance and it was all about survival. Somehow, slowly, over the years, I had completely lost who I truly was.

'In time, Luke, you are going to discover how you fill that hole and then nourish it.'

Although I struggled to completely understand what Richard meant, he was striking a chord with me. I could understand the concept that someone, in this case me, would only look for outside affirmation for their own self-worth because they weren't truly comfortable with themselves and what was inside. Richard asked me if I had ever met people who seemed to have a real peace about them. People who wouldn't feel the need to play up to the crowd in a social environment and seemed really confident in themselves – not in an arrogant way, but in a calm way.

'Yeah, I have, actually.'

'And what did you think of them?'

'Weird. I just couldn't get my head around them.'

And that was it. I found people with that peace and lack of need for affirmation weird. I actually attacked them because they intimidated me. I knew they knew something I didn't and had something I didn't, which made me uncomfortable. So, my answer to it was that they were weird because they weren't like me.

It actually made me think back to times in my career when I was critical of people who weren't like me. A good friend of mine now is my former Lancashire CCC teammate Kyle Hogg – a brilliant bloke and an outstanding cricketer. But when we played together there was sometimes this tension between us, and that was my fault. Kyle couldn't have been more different to me. I was intense, he was relaxed; I had limited ability, he was very naturally gifted; I was concerned about what everyone thought about me, and Kyle couldn't care less what other people thought. I didn't embrace how he was different to me, I shunned it. If Kyle failed then I was quick to tell myself and others why he failed, which in essence was that he didn't have enough of certain personality traits. The hidden caveat was that I had those 'necessary' traits. I couldn't embrace that he was just a different character to me. They weren't his failings, they were my failings. It was like co-existing with a big ego and a low self-worth. I'm embarrassed about that now, but it was such a good example of how I felt I needed to operate in order to survive.

It was like I believed I was the director of the show and everyone had to do what I said. If they wanted to do it a different way, then I attacked them for it. And if the show went badly, then it was their fault, not mine.

Yet I was a child who had travelled the world and seen difference everywhere. Different cultures, different lands, different colours, different food – I loved difference. Gladys, my amazing housekeeper in Peru, was different to me but I didn't feel or see any bad in that. Somehow as an adult, I had completely lost my way. Suddenly difference was a threat I couldn't stomach. It said everything about where I was at.

'But what does this have to do with drinking or any other issues?'

'It has everything to do with it, Luke. It is the essence of it. The ways in which you are acting out are just the final symptom of your underlying issues. Sort the underlying issues and you will never have to act out again.'

His words felt life-changing. I just didn't yet know how that life change would play out.

***

Richard regularly challenged us in sessions. He would often go after the biggest challenger in the group that day. He would almost bait them to challenge him and then off he would go. He was fearless about it and I often used to wonder how he hadn't been sparked out.

I actually started to really look forward to his sessions. I knew they would be interesting, and I loved the light bulb moments he was giving me. During those second two weeks I was at the hospital, every day felt like I was moving a mountain. I was understanding more and more about what I was, what I needed to do and that I had a long road ahead.

One day, Richard stormed into the room and wrote 'GOD' on the board and asked us what it meant to us. Various expletives started being shouted out:

'Don't start this shit with us.'

'Fucking load of bullshit.'

'I knew this was all a religious cult thing.'

My answer was, 'Irrelevant'. Richard jumped all over that and asked me to explain more. I immediately regretted having said something that had now brought the attention on me. It was a bit like my 'Being successful' answer; I didn't really give it much thought and just blurted out what I thought of straight away. Suddenly I was desperately trying to work out why I had said that.

'I guess because I think we're all in control of our own destiny. The word God sort of pisses me off. It's irrelevant. God is irrelevant, we are in control.'

'But I'm guessing you sort of believe in God?'

'Well yeah, I guess so, but he's not in control.'

Sadly, to Richard, this was like a red rag to a bull. I also was struggling with what I was saying and could hear the contradiction in my mind. I believed in God but felt God had no relevance in our lives. So, what exactly did I think God was doing?

'Ah, so this is about control. You believe you are completely in control of your own life.'

'Yes.'

'So, everything that happens in your life is in your control.'

'Well … yes, I guess so.'

'So, what happened when Nia died then?'

I was shocked that Richard just brought up Nia's name like that. I could feel myself getting hot. I was uncomfortable and getting cross.

'What the fuck has that got to do with it?'

'Well, you told me that you were in control of everything in your life. I know you were devastated when Nia died, so how have you reconciled that event if you believe you control everything?'

I just didn't have an answer. It was a question and a concept that was completely at odds with how I had grown to believe I operated in the world. I felt I was the master of my own destiny but how then did I explain what had happened to Nia? It was an accident, which meant things happened in the world that I didn't control ... but I had to be in control.

Richard quickly pointed out that he wasn't raising the concept of God to see if we believed in something called God. He raised the subject to see what people's reactions were. Why did everyone react so strongly and so aggressively? Whether you believe in God or not is entirely up to you, so why did everyone, including me in the end, get really defensive about it? It was a really good question.

I found it a fascinating discussion and a huge eye-opener. The discussion was not about God per se, it was about control. Why were we all so obsessed by control? I could completely relate to it. I could see how I wanted to control everything in my life and when something didn't work, it was never my fault. Even when entering The Priory, my feelings were that things would get better for me if people just started doing what I said.

I was obsessed with what people thought of me. It was a full-time job trying to maintain this level of control in my life. It was exhausting. And the great irony was that when I started drinking, I didn't have any control.

I could recognise that many of my mental health problems stemmed from this as well. My anxiety was hand in hand with my obsession to control every outcome. I even had a theory that the more I worried about something, the more likely it would fix itself. It was completely bonkers. I had the same obsession about practice at times, which no doubt had some benefits, but it was, in essence, crazy.

I had no natural outlet in my life. I was a pressure cooker constantly building up with a self-imposed need for control. Richard explained that eventually that pressure cooker would blow. In my case that would mean a binge. A binge to escape the pressure I was placing on myself. A binge to escape from myself. It was a relief getting out of my head at times.

'So, how do we let go of control?'

'A start is to ask for help from someone else.'

It was all so simple yet so elusive.

'But who is "someone else", for fucks sake?'

'It can be anyone – a friend, a group of people, a god, a tree, whatever you want. Just not you. If you can accept that your thinking has been off, then how do you think you are going to think your way out of this? The answer is, you're not. You need help from someone or something bigger than you. To truly ask and accept help, then you have to let go of believing you control everything.'

It was all just words but so powerful in mind. I could see it. I could see what Richard was talking about. To truly accept help, you had to let yourself be vulnerable. Remove the barrier of your ego and start getting honest. You had to accept that you couldn't control everyone and every outcome, and humble yourself to ask for help. Our group was basically a collection of fuck-ups and most of the time we spent complaining about the food or the water pressure. It was all so back to front. Our egos led with everything and underneath we were people who really needed help. Richard was trying to break down that barrier.

Bringing up Nia's name was a classic Richard tactic. He knew it would upset me, but he also knew *how* it would upset me. It didn't affect me from a grief point of view; it affected me from a guilt point of view. It was tapping into a part of my psyche that wanted to find peace with the whole thing but wasn't prepared to look at myself honestly in the process. He was shocking me, so I would consider the point he was making. It was all part of the process of my understanding that the work that needed to be done was on me and no one else.

As with all of Richard's sessions, the discussions could go on forever. There were always people who spent the whole session arguing with him, but he was a master at putting them back in their place. The concept of control was fascinating to me. Without exception, everyone whom I had met in The Priory was a control freak of some sorts. We were literally obsessed by it.

It created such a difficult push and pull effect in my mind. I felt like I was on the edge of the cliff. I had survived in the adult world so far by hyper-focussing on control and I was now being told that to get better, I had to learn how to let go of control. I was basically being told that to change my life, I needed to completely let go of what my concept of me was. That was truly terrifying. Questions bounced around in my head non-stop:

If this isn't me, then who am I?

Maybe I should just stick with what I know?

If I start to become all happy-clappy, will any of my good personality traits come with me?

What will people think of me?

It was really tough but I knew what I had to do. I couldn't go back to living the way I had been. I was killing myself and making everyone around me unhappy. I felt toxic. I had to find another way and I felt like I was completely out of excuses. Now was the time to change. I didn't know exactly how I was going to do this or where it was going to take me, but I needed to put on my big boy pants and find out.

I knew that I truly needed to start to listen.

I needed to get honest with myself.

I needed to become aware of my actions and my thought processes.

I needed to rediscover exactly who I was.

Chapter 9

In my last seven days at The Priory I could genuinely sense that my life was going to change forever.

In the grand scheme of things, twenty-eight days in one place doesn't seem that long, but in The Priory it felt like so much longer. It was intense – long days and a huge outpouring of emotion every day. I felt like my eyes were being truly opened. I didn't know all the answers, but I felt like I had a starting point. I felt like there was a solution to untangle myself from the knot I had got into.

I had hope.

And my hope came from a new awareness as to who I was and what I had been doing. As my first sponsor, Roy, said to me, 'You will do better when you know better. And you'll know better when you do better.'

The trap that I had fallen into was the result of an ingrained pattern of behaviour that was never going to solve my problems. Alongside this I had an unshakeable ego and a conviction that I knew better than anyone else and didn't need help. It was a toxic combination.

For the first time I could see some possibility that there was a different way to do life.

***

During my time in The Priory I worked through the early steps that were going to help me start my journey towards changing my life. This work, written and verbal, was a combination of building self-awareness and an understanding that this was about action. And that action had to come from me. It was time to gain awareness, accept responsibility and make changes. It was daunting and exhilarating at the same time.

As always, all your work was shared with the rest of the group and feedback was encouraged by your peers. I now knew that I couldn't do this all on my own and interaction with my group peers was an important step for me in asking for and accepting outside help.

I was asked, as everyone was, to write an action plan. This plan was basically a written commitment of what I felt I needed to do when I left The Priory in order to continue my recovery. I had to document things such us which support groups I would access, what my living arrangements were and how I would handle returning to work. This was the time when the reality that I would soon be back in the outside world hit me. It was a really strange feeling.

I had become so used to the routine and structure of The Priory. I was constantly supported and had no real stresses. Suddenly I faced the prospect of dealing with day-to-day life. And I needed to take into account the mayhem I had caused family and friends before I had gone in. That was all waiting for me. I felt ready but nervous.

I had one nagging question in my mind during that last week, which I decided to talk about to a therapist separately from group sessions. I had clearly suffered with some mental health issues. Before going into The Priory, there were times when I had been engulfed by a mixture of anxiety and depression. My anxiety was absolutely suffocating and would see me sitting in my shower in my flat for over an hour, terrified about having to get out and take on the day. My depression came in the form of waves of such crashing lows that nothing mattered in my world: my family, my cricket, life itself … literally nothing mattered to me at that time. In fact, sometimes the only way I could get out of it would be to plan my next night out. It would give me a temporary high and pull me out of the low.

So, I sat with Caroline, one of the therapists.

'Do you think that I have suffered with mental health issues because of my drinking or do I drink the way I do because of my mental health issues?'

I couldn't work out what was cause and what was effect. It felt a really important issue to me. I wanted to know what was leading what.

'The truth is, Luke, that you need a long period of sobriety to work this out, but what I would say, having heard everything you have told us while you've been here, is that you have never drunk alcohol normally.'

Caroline was right. I had never had a successful relationship with alcohol. I had pretended I had. God, I had really pretended I had! But it was never normal, and it was rarely successful. It almost always led to me behaving in a way I was ashamed of and/or waking up the next day crippled with anxiety. There had been times over the years that my drinking had been more 'normal', but slowly, over time, it had escalated in a negative way.

What was clear for me was that my drinking was not helping my mental health at all. This was another hugely important connection in my mind. It related to that attitude I had when I first arrived at The Priory that, *If you had my problems then you would drink like I do*. I was examining whether it was perhaps not my drinking that was to blame but my mental health.

I was now truly understanding what this was about. Drinking alcohol was destroying my life whether through mental health or any other way. But it was my choice to drink it. My choice. My responsibility. And therefore, my change to make.

I knew I had to make changes.

***

One of the other significant pieces of work I had to do in that final week was to write a letter to myself. As ever, it was to be read out in front of the group. It was such a profound piece of work for me to do. I spent a lot of time thinking about what to write but in the end just wrote what came naturally to me. The letter didn't take me that long to write in the end. Sadly, I burnt that letter immediately afterwards with some of my group mates. It was our version of a 'letting go' ceremony!

But I remember every single word I wrote to myself:

Hi Luke,

Enough.
Enough of you.
Enough of what you have been doing to my life and everyone around me.
Enough of not taking responsibility.
Enough of living in the past and the future.
Enough of hiding your shame.
Enough of being afraid to change.
Enough of feeling like I am chained to you.
Enough of believing that you are the best version of me.
Enough of secrets.
Enough of believing that you know best.
Enough of you.

I know you haven't given up yet and will try your ways again on me, but I promise you that I don't want you and am going to do everything I can to keep you away from me.

Thank you for the lessons you have taught me but enough is enough.

The truest version of Luke Sutton.

I cried as I read it to my group as a huge wave of relief swept over me. I was being a witness to the person that I had been when I walked into The Priory. I didn't want to be that person any more. I knew that I had taken the first few steps on a journey that would probably never end, but I felt committed to it. I didn't want to go back to the old version of me.

My thank you to my old self for the lessons that he had taught me was a difficult one. I knew I hadn't got anywhere near to forgiving myself for some of my behaviour, and certainly didn't feel grateful for me. So making that thanks felt a little forced, but it was me trying to make a commitment that that was how I needed to see my past. I needed to thank it for the lessons it had taught me. I knew that this was going to be a work in progress.

***

There was one other big thing that happened in my last week.

A new patient had arrived at the hospital and he was the talk of the place.

He only appeared at night and would venture out of his room to smoke outside on his own before shuffling back to his room. In basic terms, he looked like your archetypal tramp. He had a long scruffy beard and his hair was dirty and overgrown. His clothes looked equally dirty and a funny mixture of items put together, exactly as a tramp would wear from what they had picked up on the streets. He wore Timberland boots with no laces and walked hunched over and incredibly slowly. He looked in real pain. He never looked or spoke a word to anyone. The only aspect of him that looked completely out of place with his tramp look was that he wore a big expensive watch. From a distance, it looked like a big Rolex.

We would huddle around at meal and break times and talk about who this guy might be. Various ridiculous rumours went around. At one point, someone claimed he was Jason Orange from Take That. No one actually knew. We all wondered whether he would ever join us in group session.

It came to my very last day at The Priory.

Your last day tended to be focused a little around you in the group sessions of that day. You would be asked to share how you were feeling about leaving and go back over your plans to cope with the outside world.

So it came to my very last group session at The Priory.

As we sat there waiting for the therapists to walk in, the 'tramp man' shuffled in and sat down in the chair next to me. He didn't look at anyone and didn't say anything. There was a shock amongst the group after all the gossiping we had been doing. No one knew quite what to say.

He absolutely stank, and I can hand on heart say that to this day, I have never seen someone alive look so physically poorly. The whites of his eyes were completely yellow, and his face was full of sores and marks. He looked like he hadn't eaten properly for a long while as his clothes completely swamped him. But, most importantly, he looked dead inside. There was no life in his eyes. He looked completely broken as a human being.

Our therapist, Caroline, walked in.

'Hi everyone, this session is obviously going to be largely dedicated to Luke as he leaves us very shortly, but before we do that, I would like to introduce you all to Jonathan.'

He was called Jonathan.

Caroline turned to him.

'Hi Jonathan, I hope you're feeling OK. I know it's not the first time we have seen you here, so maybe you could tell the group what has happened to you to come back here?'

Jonathan's eyes engaged with Caroline, but it looked like it took a huge effort from him to actually speak. To start with he just coughed and spluttered but eventually he spoke very slowly and quietly:

'Hi Caroline, nice to see you again. You know, I was doing OK. I had stopped drinking and things were good with my wife again. I had started working again and I felt like this time it would all be different. Anyway, the wife asked me if I wanted to go on holiday with her and the boys in Wales. I was basically banned from going before this. I was so happy, you know, so I thought I best take some alcohol with me because I knew it would be quite stressful being with my wife. I had a plan.'

He would stop and struggle for his words every so often. The speed at which he spoke never got more than crawling pace.

'My plan was to drink three quarters of a bottle of vodka each day and I had measured out enough to cover all seven days. I knew that with that amount of vodka, no one would notice, and I would be fine. But then it all went fucking wrong.'

You could have heard a pin drop in the room.

'Everything was going fine but then I stupidly drank a bit too much on day two, which meant I started drinking into the other days and then completely ran out by day four. I was so stupid. I had a really good plan and I just needed to fucking stick to it. Anyway, when I ran out, I went to the local off-licence and bought more. A lot more. I drank a bottle of vodka on the way back and, of course, they noticed when I got back. Anyway, my wife went mad and packed the car up and drove the boys home.'

He was absolutely devastated. Tears started to roll from his eyes and he couldn't talk any more. Caroline seemed to want him to talk, though.

'And what happened then, Jonathan?'

'I don't really remember. I was locked out and basically carried on drinking. I know I've been on the streets for a few weeks. I'm just so annoyed with myself. If I just stick to my plans, then all will be fine. I just fucked it.'

This man looked genuinely close to death. He was your park bench drunk and yet he was still debating that he could drink successfully as long as he 'stuck to his plans'. I was absolutely shocked. I now knew why Caroline had wanted him to speak.

I just couldn't help myself say something to him:

'Hi Jonathan, I'm Luke. Thanks for sharing that. Jonathan, I mean this with love, but do you really think you can still drink and be OK? Have you seen yourself in the mirror?'

As I said that I felt like a bit of a prat. It was too harsh, but I just couldn't get my head around it. Jonathan stared at me blankly and said nothing. Instead he turned back to Caroline.

'I just want to be a dad to my boys. They are 10 and 13 now and they need me. I know I'm killing myself and they need me in their lives. I have to find a way of doing this.'

Caroline thanked Jonathan for his honesty and the rest of the session carried on with us talking about my imminent departure. Jonathan just sat in the chair lifeless and didn't say another word. Seeing Jonathan like that had a seismic impact on me. I was just about to leave The Priory and he was as ravaged by alcohol both mentally and physically as I had ever seen. Despite all his pain, he was still debating whether it was because of alcohol. It was total madness. I could picture his sons trying to grow up to be men and his wife battling with dealing with all of this. I truly felt terrible for all of them, including Jonathan.

As my time came to an end in The Priory, the universe placed my path to cross with Jonathan's. I don't know why but I was grateful for it. I knew I wanted to change my life. I knew I wanted to be a better person, a better father. Yet here I passed a man that also wanted all those things but couldn't see the wood for the trees. He was trapped in his old self. He thought that was him. He couldn't be a witness to that person and recognise that there was a better version of him out there.

A few weeks later, approaching Christmas, I was to find out that Jonathan had been found dead in his hotel room in Manchester. Cause of death was unknown, but he had been drinking for a number of days. Jonathan had been a successful lawyer, which explained the expensive watch. I cried as someone told me that news. I cried for his sons forever having to have Christmas without their dad. I cried for his wife having to pick up all the pieces without any support. I cried for Jonathan, trapped in a living hell without being able to see how to get out of it. It was utterly devastating.

As I left The Priory, I knew that I had an opportunity. An opportunity to change. But it was down to me. I felt emboldened but terrified. I was standing on the edge of a cliff but was now completely committed to making that leap of faith. I didn't know what was to come but I was ready to jump.

But importantly, as Jude drove me out of The Priory grounds, I knew that I never wanted to drink alcohol again.

Chapter 10

My final year of professional cricket proved to be a critical period in my life.

At the end of the 2010 season, I sensed that my time was coming to an end at Lancashire CCC. I was approaching my mid-thirties and knew the best I would probably get from the club would be a one-year contract extension. That was about right; I wasn't getting any better and my body was ageing.

I actually once heard David 'Bumble' Lloyd say that he should have retired in his early thirties. I remember thinking at the time that that sounded odd, but now, with the benefit of hindsight, I completely understand what he meant. From the age of 32/33, my game wasn't improving much. I could still compete at the highest level of domestic cricket, but I didn't feel a sense of excitement to evolve and push on with my game until I was 40. I had started to slightly switch off from the game and had moved into a survival mindset. I was hanging in there, basically. That mindset spells the beginning of the end, and it is really hard to recognise in yourself. I certainly didn't see it at the time.

I had an existing business already set up so my work path after cricket was pretty obvious, but recognising and accepting the moment that you should 'let go' of the game is a really tough one for any professional sportsperson. The game is your obsession and for many, very much including me, it is part of your persona. It was how I defined myself. I wasn't just working as a professional sportsman, I *was* a professional sportsman. It was one of the challenges I was presented with in The Priory by the likes of Richard. Remember the 'being successful' comment?

So, trying to recognise when to retire from professional sport is incredibly difficult and that is why it is forced upon 99 per cent of us. The cliff edge feelings I had in The Priory about whether I was ready to take the leap of faith to discover who I really was were very similar to the prospect of letting go of professional sport.

An opportunity came for me to return to Derbyshire CCC and sign a two-year contract. I still owned an apartment in Derby and the drive from our home in Cheshire was sixty to ninety minutes, so the whole thing wasn't impossible. I signed with the club and looked ahead to a new challenge at a club I knew well.

But the truth was, I was playing with fire.

***

At the start of 2011, I wasn't just hanging in there from a cricket career point of view; I was hanging in there on a personal level. My mental health was really poor, and my binges were more extreme than ever. The very last thing I needed to do was to get isolated in an apartment on my own and return to a place where I had suffered the most traumatic experience of my life.

But I now look back and recognise that I consciously or, more likely, subconsciously was willingly doing all of this. There was some part of me that wanted to unravel. I was in so much mental pain that I wanted to be left alone to torture myself. I wanted to go back to Derby for all the reasons why I shouldn't go back.

Of course, I had to work even harder at this time to make sure everything looked good. There was no way I could let anyone know how much I was struggling. If someone else recognised it then that meant I had to recognise it! As a senior player and eventually captain, that was relatively easy for me to control and manipulate, but I was actually breaking. Our preseason tour to Barbados was a perfect reflection on this. On the one hand, I was training and competing as hard as I could, and on the other, my nights out reflected the absolute opposite of this professionalism. I woke up one morning on the beach slumped against a rum shack with absolutely no idea where I was. To some people this was funny, and I would laugh along, but inside I was deeply ashamed of how I was always getting into these situations without finding any way to prevent it. I knew that I had no control.

Once the season got under way, it was more of the same. I was placing increasing pressure on my marriage and just wanted to isolate myself in my apartment in Derby. To put this into context, this was the apartment that I had lived in with Nia and where I had been when I found out about her death. I was literally torturing myself. The season at the club was challenging on and off the field, but my biggest battle was with myself. My binges continued but I also started to drink on what I would consider 'normal' nights. This would generally be a bottle or so of wine. I would make myself sick in the morning to try to purge myself and be ready for the day's cricket. I really wasn't well.

I would often go to sleep in the lounge right next to the TV, which would be on full blast. I couldn't bear the silence in the apartment and the noise would strangely help me sleep. I actually still find that nowadays, to a lesser extent. And during all of this my business outside of cricket was rapidly expanding. I was placing more and more demands upon myself. I was escalating in every possible way.

I now reflect back on that last season in professional cricket and my descent in my ever-decreasing circle was now speeding up; I was approaching the bottom. My performances were OK but personally I felt desperate. I will always remember the night out after our Derbyshire CCC End-of-Season Awards. We were all in Derby city centre and I was badly drunk. I remember being in a bar and thinking I was in a place where I would know everyone. This is where Nia and all her friends were from and in my drunken haze I thought this was where I would find comfort. People would be coming up to me and asking me how I was, remembering the old times and comforting me for everything that had happened.

But there was none of that.

I was alone and a pain to be with. I annoyed people and was rude as I stumbled about. I don't really know what I was looking for but whatever it was, it didn't exist.

I wanted to live in the past because I couldn't face handling the present. It was like the reality of life had just become too painful for me to bear. Maybe it had always been that way, so my answer was to escape. That escape didn't just come in the form of alcohol; it came in the form of not being in reality. I wanted to escape from me.

My present was so painful that I thought it was easier to sit in the shit of the past. I don't even know whether I was actually missing Nia. I was just unravelling, and this was my go-to place.

I was sad, desperate and deeply lonely, and the thing getting in the way of me asking for help was … ME.

It would only take my full breakdown for me to finally be able to reach out for help.

***

So less than four weeks after leaving The Priory, I retired from professional cricket. It was absolutely the right thing to do and I am very grateful for everyone involved in that decision.

At the time, it was really difficult but it felt like a big step in my post-Priory recovery. By retiring I was giving myself space from an environment in which I had nearly destroyed myself, but also, and crucially, it was a step towards letting go of that persona I thought I was within professional cricket. Work hard, play hard, to a level of intensity few could match – that's what I thought I was for the best part of twenty years. In retiring, I was also recognising that life needed to change in order for me to find a better way to live. That persona had to die.

I didn't love my retirement press release. I mentioned difficulties in my life that I didn't need to and didn't mention any difficulties with alcohol. The reason for that is that I was still trying to make sense of how I was going to handle everything in the outside world. I needed a few months to get my head around it all, but I didn't have that time. I was club captain, and everybody needed to know where things stood. It was just a reflection of where I was at.

Despite my retirement being an easier decision than it was for other players, because I knew it was necessary and I had a way to earn a living, I was still hit by some of the many challenges sportspeople face when they leave the game they have been dedicated to. The biggest challenge, without question, was structure. I really had no idea how much structure professional cricket had put in my life. Where to be, when to play, when to train, what to eat, when to eat, what to wear, when to sleep – it is all set out for you when you play professional cricket. Suddenly, all that structure was gone. I didn't even know what time I should start my day.

Am I supposed to do 9–5 now? I had no idea.

The first time I went to the gym after my retirement I didn't know what I should do. And remember, I was a gym bunny! I loved training. But as a pro, I had always done it with the help of a strength and conditioning coach, and more often than not, that coach would literally be standing next to me as I trained. Now I was deciding how many reps to do and what would be best for me on that day. I didn't know what I was doing. It was actually really pathetic.

That battle with a sudden lack of structure actually held me in good stead in later years when, as manager of James Taylor, I had to help him cope with his immediate drop out of the game due to his heart condition. I knew that the vacuum of structure for him would be a huge challenge. I suggested we set up a Google calendar, which James and I shared, and still do. To begin with we would just put in hospital appointments or that his mum was coming around to the house. But I knew that it would represent some sort of structure for him, which is what he needed.

Life in the 'normal' world when I left The Priory was really tough. My family, and particularly Jude, gave me incredible support. I had caused chaos before going into the hospital, but they were amazing with me. At times it did feel like everyone was treading on eggshells around me, and that nervousness was totally understandable. I may have moved on in my mind from the toxic person I had been, but it wasn't that distant a memory for everyone around me. 'The jury's out' is a phrase that you could quite easily believe people were attributing to me at the time.

I attended lots of support groups and realised I had a long way to go. Some days I felt like I was making giant strides and other days like

I was wading through treacle. But I was determined to try to keep moving forward. I was surrounded by people who cared for me and that was priceless.

The one thought that remained solid in my mind was that I didn't want to drink alcohol again. Deep in my soul I knew the damage it was causing me. In the past I had pretended that it was all fun and games, but the genie was out of the bottle and there was no going back for me.

But not wanting to drink alcohol again and actually putting that into practice are two very different things. Everyone was used to me being a drinker on a night out. It was part of me. Suddenly I was changing the rules and it was weird for lots of my friends. Some didn't think it was necessary and some thought I just needed a break from it and could then get back on it. I was also trying to work and that involved going to social events where alcohol was everywhere, and I had insecurities about dealing with that social pressure. It was all new ground for me so I came up with various tactics to get through it.

Of course, as soon as you decline an alcoholic drink, you are faced with, 'Why are you not drinking?'

The easiest answer would have always been, 'Well, when I drink, I lack any sort of real control and start fucking up my life and losing my mind. So, thanks for the offer, but I'll pass.'

Sadly, you can't say that most of the time, although I wish I had done a few times! My reasons for not wanting to drink were and still are personal to me. I'm not trying to place judgement or opinion on what is and isn't a drinking problem; I just know that for me alcohol doesn't work. It doesn't bring out the best version of me, so I don't want to do it. It really is that simple. But as soon as you go against a social norm, you often find that people want to debate it with you. I'm not really sure why. I think it is because we are all so programmed to do what we are 'meant' to do, and drinking is a big part of that in the UK. As soon as you step out of that particular lane, people get nervous and interested. However, there is no debate for me; this is just what is right for me. Likewise, I don't like debating with people what is right for someone else who is trying to recover from similar problems to mine. I don't know what is right for someone else; I only know what the right recovery path for me is. I have spent too much of my life believing and pretending that I knew better than everyone else. A big part of my recovery is accepting the knowledge that I don't know any better than anyone else.

I knew then and still know now, in a place deep in my soul, what sort of path I need to take in my life, and that doesn't involve alcohol.

So, I embarked on trying to navigate through life as a non-drinker without attracting too much attention from anyone. I wanted to be 'under the radar'. However, in the first year of my retirement and sobriety I was fortunate enough to be invited by Jenny Smith to the Professional Cricketers' Association Dinner. Jenny was the lead for Jaguar's cricket sponsorship. The PCA Dinner was a classic event for me to go wild at, but now I was going as a sober man. When I got the invite I didn't want to turn it down, but I also didn't want to get myself in a difficult spot. I thought long and hard about it and in the end decided to go but emailed Jenny:

Hi Jenny,

Thanks so much for the invite and I will happily accept! Can't wait! One thing to mention though is that I might be quite boring; I can't drink on the night! I've got a kidney infection, so I need to stay off the booze. Sorry about that but really looking forward to it.

Luke x

Jenny was great about it all and after some early questioning on the night, the whole thing passed without a fuss. The old chestnut of a kidney infection came up a few times in that first year of sobriety!

Other little tricks I would use included always buying my own drinks; sometimes pretending I was drinking vodka & tonic; letting people pour me wine but then never picking up the glass; or just telling people I was having a break from the booze. It was never actually as big a deal as I made out in my mind. The lack of fuss and my surprise at that was a reflection of my abnormal relationship with alcohol. I was obsessed with what I was drinking and what everyone else was drinking. It was a big deal to me and I presumed everyone else was like that. But normal drinkers aren't like that; they couldn't really care less.

This is not to say everything went smoothly. There was one particular time when I would have buckled had not a great friend stepped in.

I was managing Jimmy Anderson and we were invited to the Professional Footballers' Association Dinner, again in my first year of sobriety. It was a big black-tie event and there was a lot of alcohol. Jimmy is like a brother to me in many ways and knew all about The Priory and my non-drinking. We sat next to each other at dinner and had a great time. Jimmy was a star attraction for a lot of footballers in the room who were secret cricket lovers. We met up with Joe Hart at the bar after dinner and the drinks were flowing. I was back in that dressing room environment of professional sport. I could feel myself buckling to try to stay with the crowd while not drinking. I wanted to be cool and popular again, and my insecurities were running riot. I wanted everyone to like me. I'd get the odd question why I wasn't drinking, and I would just try to ignore it.

From the bar, it was decided we would go to a club. I definitely didn't need to be there, but I wanted to be with Jimmy and I wanted to be part of the crowd again. The club was like the bar but worse. Everyone was drinking and dancing, and I was drinking Diet Coke. I couldn't bear it. I felt awkward. As people got drunker, I got more sober. I was boring myself at times. Eventually I couldn't take it any longer and told Jimmy I was getting a drink. Maybe I told Jimmy because I wanted him to stop me. I'll never know. But I didn't just sneak off and get a drink in a crowded club. I told him I was going to do it, which might have been a little cry for help. He was amazing.

He immediately told me to stop and think about it. Bear in mind that Jimmy had had a few drinks by now and would probably like his buddy to loosen up a bit. So it was a big thing for him to think like this. He asked me not to do it, and I didn't. It wasn't a client to manager thing; it was just a friend to friend thing. He got me to pause, which gave me enough time to realise it wasn't a good idea and it was time to get home.

***

That first year of sobriety became a first for everything while not drinking. Some of it was relatively easy and some of it was very difficult, but I got through it. When I reached 13 October 2012, I felt a huge sense of achievement and gratitude. When in The Priory, I met a friend of a fellow inmate who came in to visit. She had also been in The Priory and told me she was a year and a half without a drink. One and a half years: she might as well have said one million and a half years! It sounded so long, and I couldn't believe it. I was shocked and astounded. Yet here I was with a year of sobriety under my belt and it felt incredible.

Sobriety was giving me space in my mind to try to discover more about myself. Some of it I really didn't like, but it was giving me a chance to find the truest and best version of myself. As I discovered more, I realised I had so much further to go. The Priory had been magical but, in some ways, I had just been scratching the surface in dealing with the stress, anxiety and pressure of real life. Outside of the cocoon of The Priory bubble was where my real recovery began.

Step by step I was moving forward, sometimes slowly, sometimes quickly, but I was always moving forward. Relationships were being repaired and I was definitely being a better all-round person. I was learning to live sober.

There was just so much further for me to go.

Chapter 11

Richard was the first person who told me that I was a living pressure cooker.

I was living life the best way I knew while pressure built up inside me until ... BANG! The pressure would get too much, and I would need a release. I would need an escape from life, my mind and, basically, me. This would be acted out in the form of a binge that I couldn't control, which almost always featured alcohol. This would be followed by a feeling of shame, then a purge and recovery, then another pressure build-up, and bingo, we were back where we started!

I understand that many people have these sorts of feelings at some time in their lives – a few drinks in the pub after a long week at work or time spent with the kids is an escape in itself. It was just that my pattern of behaviour manifested itself in a much more extreme way. It was completely unsustainable and, most importantly, it was something that I couldn't live with.

Over the months and years after I had been at The Priory, I was able to work with people to get a far better understanding of who I am and how I react to life's problems. In essence it has been a journey of self-discovery and self-awareness. I don't claim to have all the answers, but I do now know much more about myself and how to live a better life.

I could never have done this on my own. I needed people around me who could show me the wood from the trees. I couldn't see it and, left to my own devices, I would eventually drift back into that unhealthy pattern of behaviour.

***

Where did that pressure within me come from?

Slowly, over a period of time, I just coped less and less well with the stresses of life. I have had some difficult things happen that exacerbated this, but my natural characteristics meant I was predisposed to these sorts of problems, and then the environment I was in brought it all to the boil. There was never one particular thing that kicked everything off; it was just me, trying to survive in the world and not being able to see any different. Importantly, all of the mistakes I made were my choices; I own them, but I recognise now that I just didn't know a better way to handle life at the time.

My strengths proved to be my weaknesses.

My ability to hyper focus on things meant that I would be extremely diligent with my work rate in and out of cricket, but it also meant that I wouldn't be able to let things go. There was no break from whatever I was obsessing about. I often describe it as trying to draw a line as straight as you can, but it is never perfect. You just keep trying. Again and again, and again.

My obsession with winning made me hugely competitive, which helped me in many ways, but it also became what I defined myself by. I didn't leave much room in my life for anything of real substance; it was all about being successful or appearing to be successful. Within that obsession, I lost who I truly was.

I was incredibly sensitive about everything, which meant that I was often able to be compassionate with others but it also meant I was obsessed with what people thought about me. Analysing the past and the future were full-time jobs for me because I was obsessed by opinion and took everything so personally.

And throughout all of this ran one big theme – control. I wanted to control everything in life. I believed that everything was in my control and it all depended on what I did and if people listened to me. That need for control was to manage all of my worries and obsessions – it was mentally exhausting.

I would hold on for so long but eventually I would need a release. This would then be coupled with an inability for me to control my drinking once I started. Almost by nature, this would lead to me behaving in ways I wasn't proud of and the inevitable shame that would follow. I would repeat that cycle so many times that eventually the only answer would be to push the shame so far down in my soul that I would stop recognising it.

And sadly, my answer to all of this was more of the same. My answer to pressure was to try to exert more control in my life, which in turn created even more pressure. It was a vicious circle.

Preseason cricket trips epitomised this. I would be anxious about the season ahead so my work rate would be at an all-time high. I would heap pressure and anxiety on myself and then eventually need a massive blowout. That would happen and then I would beat myself up over doing so and would work twice as hard in an attempt to purge myself. It would keep happening again and again.

At the same time, I would be working really hard to make sure everything looked great to the outside world and I would be in denial that I needed any help. That lack of humility to ask for help was all part of the problem. To have done so would have meant I would have to accept that I didn't have everything under control. I couldn't do that. My faith in my own control was what the whole thing was based around. I *had* to control everything.

These were all my mistakes and all my choices; I take responsibility for it all. I also know that many people, even without the extent of my problems, experience some of the things I'm talking about. It was just the escalating and extreme nature of my behaviour that made things different. As time went on I was coping less and less, and my behaviour was becoming more and more extreme. Eventually I had to fall apart entirely in order to be willing to consider a different way of doing things.

***

What was my solution?

A critical starting point was to recognise that although it wasn't healthy for me to drink alcohol, sobriety wasn't the only solution to my issues. Drinking alcohol to extreme levels was just a symptom of the mental state I was getting myself into. If I really wanted to find a solution, then stopping drinking wasn't enough; I had to deal with the reasons why I got to that point.

I have found out many things about myself during this journey, some of which have been very uncomfortable to know. One of the biggest discoveries was to realise how utterly self-obsessed I could be. It was all about me! My anxieties and obsessions were never about other people, they were always about me. There's no question that Nia's death exacerbated this because as a result I decided it was time that I took from life what I wanted, but the underlying self-obsession was always there.

I had to learn that the world wasn't there to do my bidding. I was asked in my early days of recovery to do a kind thing for someone every day and not tell them I had done it. *Not to tell them* ... I found it so hard! My whole life was so transactional that if I did something kind for someone then I would definitely want them to know so that I could accept their wonderful thanks and feel better about myself. It all sounds simple, but it was such a different way for me to look at life. I had to learn, day by day, to try to think of others before thinking of myself. And what did this have to do with pressure and drinking? Actually, a lot. By thinking of others and taking myself out of myself, I would release the pressure on myself. Suddenly my anxieties weren't as important because I wanted to give more consideration to others.

However, the biggest learning was how to let go of control. Control flowed through everything I did. It was the cornerstone of everything I believed and was always the trigger for the pressure that built up in me. It was a huge topic for me.

But if I am not in control, then who is?

It was the biggest question that kept spinning back on me. It was all well and good telling me to be less controlling, but I needed to understand how to do this differently. It's a bit like telling someone who worries a lot to stop worrying. It doesn't help. That worrier will worry by nature. They need another way of approaching the challenge they face or believe they face.

The whole 'control' subject always took me back to that session in The Priory when Richard challenged us about God. We all got so defensive about it and as soon as I was told that I needed to let go of control, I immediately leapt on the presumption that this would be about God. I was going to be asked to let go of control to God. I could immediately feel myself getting defensive again about it. That reaction actually said so much about my lack of understanding of control – as well as my lack of understanding about faith.

I was like a baby learning to walk with all these hugely fundamental thoughts in my life. Why was I so defensive about God? Why did I perceive that it was either me or God that controlled everything? I started to understand that my perception of God and faith was really narrow, and it all led back to me wanting to believe that I could and should control everything. My perception of God and faith was a direct challenge to this, and so, my only response was to attack it.

Early on in recovery, I had strong people around me who showed me a different way to look at this whole subject. They asked me to consider what I was most afraid of in the world – failure and judgement being the biggest two things.

The failure was what I felt if I didn't get something right, however big or small. It might be dropping a catch to lose a televised match or getting a question wrong in front of everyone at the pub quiz.

Judgement was what people thought about me and this was intrinsically linked to failure. What if people didn't like me … thought I was stupid … thought I was boring … or wasn't good enough?

I was asked to consider that I was not in total control of either of these outcomes – my failure or other people's judgement. For example, I could do everything perfectly in a business negotiation, but someone simply changed their mind, for reasons out of my control, and the deal didn't happen. I could practise as hard as I could on a particular skill but on the day, someone was just better than me. I could be the best person I could be, but someone might still not like me. What if I was just a little spec on the earth and everything was being sorted out in the big universe and all I had to do was be the best I could be?

All I had to do was be the best I could be.

I was being asked to consider the concept that all I had to do was be the best version of myself at any given moment and leave the outcome to be sorted by the universe. I was being asked to stop focusing on outcomes and simply think about being the best I could be. It was so simple.

So simple!

But this was profoundly different to how I had been looking at the world up till now. All I had focused on were the outcomes – would I win, would people like me, what if this happens or if that happens? I was now being asked to concentrate on the present: be the best I could be NOW and leave the rest to take care of itself. It was so subtle yet so powerful. I was starting to understand the concept of living in the now.

And how did it all make me feel? RELIEVED!

I had spent my whole life worrying about outcomes and suddenly I realised that all I needed to do was be the best I could be at any given moment and leave the outcome to be what it would be, and that was ALWAYS enough. It was complete relief. I didn't need to worry about what might or might not happen; I just needed to concentrate on the now. It was truly like a weight off my shoulders.

And I was warned that every time I felt uneasy or anxious it was because I had stepped out of this thought process. I would likely be stressing about the future and have fallen back into a belief that I could fully control the outcome. I would have fallen out of living in the now.

Suddenly I had a whole new concept of control and faith, and really it had nothing to do with God – unless I wanted it to. It was simply that I accepted I wasn't fully in control of outcomes and, more so, that all I needed to do was concentrate on being the best I could be at any given moment.

It was so simple, but earth-shattering for me. However, this would need practice. It wouldn't feel natural to me. I needed to practise it every day because without paying attention to it I would slip back to my old way of thinking. It was just an extraordinary change for me.

Aligned with all of this was also the question of how I would deal with my hypersensitivity. I took everything so personally and was very sensitive to what anyone said or what I thought they had said about me. I could overreact to anything and it all contributed to the pressure that built up inside me.

I was asked to examine why I was so sensitive to what someone thought about me. It wasn't just what my mother thought about me, it was what anyone thought about me! The answer was so simple again. I had really lost any true feeling of self-worth. The entire basis of what I thought about myself depended on what other people told me. I constantly looked for outside affirmation because I had no internal recognition of it. The more I looked out, the less and less I had within me to reconcile how I was doing as a person. The best example of this was if I had a disagreement with someone, on a big or a small scale. That person would live in my head non-stop for days, weeks ... maybe forever because I couldn't let go of the fact that they disagreed with me and might not like me. I would obsess about them and the argument we had had. I would talk to anyone I could about it to convince them that I was right and they were wrong. I could not let it go. And why?

It was because someone disagreeing with me or not liking me was a direct pointer, in my mind, that I wasn't enough as a person. I didn't have enough self-worth to respect their opinion on the matter and myself and walk away. I couldn't do that because I was entirely reliant on other people telling me how I should value myself, and I believed that this person was telling me that I wasn't good enough. In my mad mind, for me to accept their opinion would be like accepting that I wasn't enough. It was all completely back to front. As always, my only answer would be to attack that person as a form of defence.

So, the answer lay in discovering who I really was and building up my own self-worth, while simultaneously arresting that habit of constantly looking for outside affirmation. The answers always lay within me. This was an inside job. But this was going to be a lengthy process. In the same way an unhealthy pattern of behaviour can gradually cause everything to deteriorate, a healthy one can slowly rebuild everything. I had to go back to that mantra of simply concentrating on being the best I could be at any given moment. With every moment I did the next right thing, I would be slowly rebuilding my self-worth. I would always remember Richard's words when he asked me if I had ever heard of the saying 'having a hole in your soul'. I fully understood him now. The hole was a lack of self-worth and understanding of who you really were.

But I was now filling that hole in my soul, slowly but surely, and was surrounded by like-minded people who could help guide me through this growth. An early discovery for me was that I am actually quite an introvert rather than an extrovert. As far as I could remember, I had always believed myself to be an extrovert who loved people and parties. But the extrovert in me only appeared when I drank alcohol and was who I became after a few drinks. My true character is very quiet and would much prefer a quiet night in than being surrounded by people in a bar.

*****

I am acutely aware that as I write all of this it sounds like it is information and knowledge that I simply needed to learn and then all would be fine … a bit like a piece of coursework. That's just not true.

I was learning a different way to live life. Not for a day but for the rest of my life. And my old patterns of behaviour were deeply ingrained, so it has been a continuous learning experience.

I have got it wrong on many occasions, but over time I have learnt to get it right more often. Most importantly, I now had a design for living that gave me a path to try to stay on. There was no end point on this path, just a track to try to stick to.

Over a period of time, I had gone from feeling alone, desperate and without any actual solutions, to feeling like I had a real chance to live the rest of my life happy and free. I now had a way of life that could mean I didn't have a pressure build-up in my mind and I didn't need an escape from life or from myself. I could sit in the reality and beauty of life.

My past mistakes were all my responsibility but now my greatest responsibility was to live a better life.

I now had a chance of finding peace in my life.

Chapter 12

Ｉt is becoming more and more apparent that professional sport is a breeding ground for addictive behaviour.

Since retiring from my playing career, I have begun managing a number of high-profile sportspeople and have been able to view the world of professional sport from a different angle. When you're in the middle of it, it is very difficult to get a clear understanding of the environment in which young professional sportsmen and women live. I can now look in from the outside but with enough inside information to get a much better perspective on it.

To be successful in professional sport you have to have addictive traits. You need to be hyperfocused, obsessive, a control freak, self-obsessed and also perhaps to carry some fear of failure within you. Those were many of the characteristics that I had to front up to in order to rebuild my life, yet they had helped me survive in professional sport for nearly two decades. They are essential for anyone to survive and thrive at high levels of sport.

Add to this the euphoric nature of performing, let alone succeeding, in front huge audiences, as well as the outside affirmation and adoration that sports stars receive and can then come to crave. It seems therefore ridiculous that we wonder why so many sportspeople suffer addictive behaviour problems during their careers, and possibly even more so after their careers have ended.

Another important factor to add to the mix that has infiltrated the professional sporting world and indeed the world in general in the last five to ten years is social media. When I started as a professional cricketer, we would more often than not go to the clubhouse bar after a day's play for a drink with teammates and the opposition. It meant we would talk to each other. It is different now. The first thing most players do as soon as they are allowed to after a day's play is check their phones. They are then head down and locked into Instagram, WhatsApp, Twitter and the rest of it. They don't talk to each other as players have done in the past.

I know a number of head coaches across professional cricket and they all agree that one of their biggest challenges nowadays is to find leaders. Finding a potential captain of a team is like gold dust and yet ten years ago, there were often four or five senior players competing within the team for the captaincy. Because this generation largely communicates with each other via social media, it doesn't create an environment in which natural leaders are born. Leaders are found in environments where players speak openly and honestly to each other. They rise up from the pack and show themselves as someone willing to take charge. There isn't that sort of communication in dressing rooms any more. I was very lucky to share a dressing room with Stuart Law for six years and he would let you know in no uncertain terms what needed to be done on the field. It didn't matter whether he was captain or not, he was a leader of men.

So, the question is, why does this relate to potential addictive behaviour issues for players? Well, my overriding emotions throughout all my troubles were loneliness and shame. I isolated my thoughts from everyone because I didn't think anyone thought like me or had the same issues as me. I was embarrassed about who I truly was. I didn't want to reach out because it would mean I would have to face everything. I kept digging a deeper and deeper hole for myself, which in the end meant there was no escape other than me completely breaking down. If the influence of social media now means that players are isolating their thoughts more and more, then that is a very dangerous situation.

Professional sportspeople are often seen as 'lucky' or 'privileged', and in many ways they are. But also in that group are young people whose issues turn them into ticking time bombs. In my opinion, there has never been a greater time for professional sportspeople to be carefully watched and supported.

***

As news breaks that a young sportsperson has got into trouble in a nightclub or in some other drink-related incident, the overwhelming reaction of people is 'What an idiot!', 'Doesn't he know how lucky he is?' or 'Why doesn't he just keep his head down?' And of course, there is always a strong element of idiocy involved, but I wish people would take the time to look at why these things happen.

I narrowly avoided drink-related incidents throughout my career and maybe I was lucky that I wasn't that high profile. I was regarded by many as a model professional and not as an idiot who took for granted what I had. But it could have all happened to me. So, I think that is a really easy stick to throw at a young sportsperson when you haven't taken the time to really understand them and their environment.

Many of these people are living pressure cookers, just like I was, and they know they need to 'keep their head down' and that they are 'very lucky', but they also crave a release from the pressure at some point. And the higher profile that person is, then the higher the tendency for them to be feeling the pressure.

This doesn't mean that I think drink or drug-related incidents are acceptable. When I saw Ben Stokes's fight in the streets of Bristol, I was as shocked as anyone, but I also took time to think about him and the space in which he lives. Heaping shame upon someone will not help them in the long run. We need to understand them as a person, be wary of warning signs they may show and then support them as much as possible to avoid a blow-up happening. When someone like Ben leaves the game, they will need just as much, if not more, support.

During the writing of this book, two news stories within cricket have broken. Two different stories, yet worth comparison in the context of this book. Firstly, Alex Hales allegedly failed a second test for recreational drugs and was subsequently dropped from all the England Cricket squads. Secondly, Robin Smith published his outstanding autobiography detailing his battle with alcoholism. The reaction to both stories and individuals from the media, ex-players and public couldn't have been more different. Before I expand on this, it's worth pointing out that I believe the correct decision was made in dropping Alex from the England squads. Alex has been treated, by and large, with considerable judgment. Even when talk started over whether he should be called up to the England World Cup squad because of injury, it was openly discussed whether he would compromise the 'values of the team'. He was affectively being labelled as an overindulgent and stupid young man. On the other hand, Robin has been treated with complete sympathy and admiration for his bravery and honesty in dealing with his problems. I agree with the reaction to Robin, but I would challenge you to give this comparison more thought.

Alex and Robin played cricket in different eras. Robin's cricketing era was definitely one of 'work hard, play hard'. Alex's cricketing era is one which is more professional in that sense. By his own admission, Robin was a big partier during his playing days. With the attention as it is on England players now and the advent of social media, it is not unfair to say that Robin could have found himself in more trouble if he was an England player today. I'm certainly not suggesting Robin would have failed a drugs test, but what if he had got into alcohol related trouble? What would we have labelled him as? I'm also not suggesting that Alex goes on to have the problems that Robin has experienced, but we need to consider whether we are happy to label people 'overindulgent' when we don't recognise the problems being shown in an earlier stage of a process. Yet when it has reached a place of total crisis, e.g. Paul Gascoigne, or of recovery, e.g. Robin Smith, we label it much more sympathetically.

Don't get me wrong, someone in Alex's shoes needs the shock of being dropped and hearing some home truths, but simply shaming someone to 'teach them a lesson' could be missing a bigger point. I believe that we have to recognise the possibility that a process may be underway which needs careful attention now, rather than wait for it to reach a crisis point before we throw out a few fairly meaningless sympathetic tweets.

I also believe that gambling is the silent killer amongst many sportspeople. Drinking involves the risk of being seen in public. It also damages fitness levels, which are now constantly measured. There is enough to put a sportsperson off from doing it, whereas gambling can be done very much under the radar and still gives that release and buzz. Professional sportspeople don't have to gamble on their own sport – indeed, it is illegal – because there is a plethora of other sports for them to choose from. It can all be done online so no one can see what they are doing. And they often have enough readily available cash to get started. It can be completely private and, as a result, very dangerous.

I read about Joey Barton's addition to gambling when it became public and I wasn't overly shocked. He was someone who had already dealt with drinking issues so to hear that gambling had become a problem for him didn't surprise me. Joey is a person who polarises opinion, with possibly more haters than supporters. As a result, there was a flood of 'What an idiot!' type of comments. Joey actually wrote a really interesting article in the media about the whole thing, not absolving himself of blame, but pointing out that the amount of gambling advertising within football didn't help someone like himself. If someone took the time to consider Joey as a person and the environment in which he operated, then I believe they could gain a better perspective on it and be less inclined to throw a careless insult at him.

I spent an English winter playing club cricket in Perth, Australia. My parents subsequently bought a house there, so I went back to Perth a number of times. Throughout my time there, the Australian Rules Footballer Ben Cousins was the big news. Ben's story has always been one I have been a little bit obsessed by.

Ben was basically what every professional sportsman wanted to be. Maybe what every guy wanted to be. He was exceptional at Aussie Rules, the most popular of all Australian sports. He was a young captain of the West Coast Eagles and led them to the Premiership win in 2006. He also won the Brownlow Medal in 2005 as the most valuable player in the league. He was handsome, with a Baywatch-style body. He was enigmatic, charismatic and idolised by many, including myself. Most importantly, Ben was a warrior on and off the field. His intensity to training was infamous. He trained harder than anyone else and pushed himself to levels that left others looking on in amazement. His fitness was off the charts and his work rate during games extremely difficult to match. It was his sheer intensity in the sport that was extraordinary.

But he had the same intensity off the field. His partying was legendary. Perth is a small place and he was king. He partied harder than anyone else and was loved for it. People simply wanted to be Ben Cousins.

I look back on it all now with real sadness.

Suddenly Ben's incidents with the police started to mount up. And they started to escalate in nature. The league's administrators and the club coaches didn't know what to do with him. He was an exceptionally talented young man and they all just wanted him to be back playing 'footy'. The fans demanded it as well. But trouble followed him and so he was constantly treated with a mixture of scorn or appeasement. In my opinion, there was little understanding of why he was acting the way he was.

Commentators of the sport didn't know what to say about him. Many came out with the old lines of 'He needs to remember how lucky he is' and 'He's just a spoilt young man'. In hindsight, the lack of understanding of someone showing addictive behaviour patterns was astonishing. And in the middle of it was Ben doing his best to pretend he had everything in hand; it was his family who were crumbling around him. The problem was that Ben didn't look like an 'addict'. He was handsome and an incredible physical specimen. He wasn't a park bench drunk or drug addict in a drug den. So people couldn't place him, and they therefore couldn't really understand him. His family did everything they could, but Ben just wasn't capable of recognising the help he truly needed. Most importantly, he was still playing his sport. He was still in the environment that encouraged every characteristic in him that made him exceptional on the field … and was killing him off the field.

Ben Cousins' story is long and painful and will be told to future generations to come. A guy who had it all but whose life has now fallen apart. His time is now split between court, rehab and jail. His looks have gone and there is absolutely no doubt what he has become. Commentators now confidently label him a 'chronic drug addict' because he looks the part, but what about before? What about when he was called 'spoilt' and needed 'to keep his head down'; what was he then? The same people comment that he clearly isn't taking in what he needs to in rehab in order to get better. And that may be the case, but why are they saying that now and not before? It is simply because he now looks like the drug addict that they perceive.

We are in a time when more than ever before there needs to be greater understanding of addictive behaviour patterns amongst professional sportspeople. Let us try to support the likes of Ben Cousins *before* he looks bad enough to fit our perception of an 'addict'. There were enough warning signs, but the emphasis has to be less about 'How do we get this guy back on the field asap?' and more, 'We might have a long-term issue with this guy that we need to start talking to him and educating him about now.' Whether people like to admit it or not, the attention is geared more towards what a person's performance is on the field of play. If that person is playing well and seemingly happy and having fun off the field, then as long as they don't get into trouble, all is considered OK.

That is simply not good enough.

Professional sporting clubs and governing bodies seem intent on ignoring warning signs and papering over cracks to hopefully get an athlete through their playing career without an issue. But that can lead to an individual harbouring a problem that can then escalate and cause immeasurable problems. In Ben's case it all unravelled while he was playing. For Paul Gascoigne, it unravelled in his retirement, but it is the same process.

Gazza was possibly the most gifted British footballer of his generation and now is a tragic figure who we all hope will get better. He is a shadow of his former self. But do we honestly think that there were no warning signs while he was playing? Of course there were. But while he was playing brilliantly and being Gazza off the field, it was all fun and giggles. People just enjoyed the ride while they could and yet now mutter, 'What ever happened to Paul Gascoigne?' The warning signs were just too boring for us to pay attention to. We are all responsible to some extent for fuelling the persona that was and is 'Gazza' – the Geordie lad who was a clown off the field and brilliant on it, with whom we all loved to laugh. But sadly, as we all moved our attention on to the next sporting star, Gazza was left as Gazza, trapped in a persona that he can't get out of ... doing what he has always done and hoping for a different result.

I was extremely fortunate to have been a teammate of Andrew 'Freddie' Flintoff and equally fortunate to call him a friend. Freddie has been really honest about his own journey with alcohol, having given it up a few years ago, and I admire him hugely for this. It is all well and good someone of my profile battling through it, but being someone as high profile as Freddie or Gazza presents an even greater mountain to climb. I largely put that down to the persona that needs to be broken through. As with the 'Gazza' persona, there was also the 'Freddie Flintoff' persona – the legend on the field taking on the Australians, and the hilarious drunk at Downing Street and the Trafalgar Square celebrations having spent the night drinking the bar dry. We loved him for it ... and we all wanted to be him. There is a public expectation for that persona to play the act and that individual feels that expectation. The Gazzas and the Freddies can feel a burden to play up to that act because that is what they believe everyone loves them for. That is who they believe they are. If you have become so dependent on outside affirmation, as I had, then letting go of that persona you believe you are is excruciatingly difficult. I remember Freddie's early days on the TV show *A League of Their Own*. He was openly referred to as 'the drunk'. Others on the show had their personas but that was Freddie's, whether he liked it or not. Freddie has managed to break away from that persona and the enormity of that personal achievement should not be underestimated. We now see the real Andrew Flintoff – talented, creative, empathetic, calm and hilarious, and a true family man. Tragically, we might not ever see that happen in Gazza. He is still 'Gazza'.

This isn't about labelling people as addicts. I don't think such labels are very helpful; they just make people overtly analyse whether or not they are an addict. But we all perceive what an addict looks like in different ways. I once told a family member that to solve some of my issues, it wasn't just about stopping drinking. It was more than just about the booze. He just looked at me completely perplexed and replied, 'Of course, it is about the booze. Someone with these problems just needs to stop drinking.'

I don't judge him for his opinion and instead I now use it as a reminder that amongst us there are many different perceptions of what an addict looks like. With so many different perceptions then I don't think it is helpful for us to go around labelling people as if we know best. I definitely don't know best. That's why I am always at pains to describe these problems as 'addictive behaviour' rather than anything else.

Labels such as 'addict' or 'alcoholic' can often be used to shame someone in public and that will never help them with their issues. They are already burying enough of their own self-created shame, and adding to that will do nothing to help. But most importantly, these labels also create unhelpful debate. Once there is a specific label used, questions start to arise like:

Is he or she really bad enough to be an alcoholic?
What is an alcoholic?
Oh, you weren't that bad!
Yeah you drink a lot but you're not an alcoholic!

People try to decide if they or others fit their own definition of an addict or alcoholic, without really knowing what it means. They also then have a marker for when they believe it is 'bad enough' to do something about it, e.g., 'When someone becomes an alcoholic then they need help'. But why is this debate even necessary? If alcohol or another sort of behaviour has a destructive influence on someone's life, then isn't that enough of a reason for them to get help for it? I feel passionately that this whole area needs to be understood so much better. The lack of knowledge leads to people dealing with issues far too late and others dealing with them with far too little compassion. Of course, if someone chooses to call themselves an addict or alcoholic, then that is different, but I am extremely wary of people placing labels on others. So I would rather avoid labels like this and just talk to people on a level that makes them feel that you understand where they are coming from. You don't judge them; you just need to support them. Help them see the wood from the trees.

***

There were times during the careers of all these people I've mentioned that we could have recognised a problem for what it was. We could have acknowledged the warning signs before their behaviour stopped being fun or we stood in judgement of them. We could have seen what they might become. We could have acted before they started to look bad enough to be in need of help.

The public and the media will pump up the highest profile people like Gazza because that is the nature of the entertainment industry. But people within professional sporting organisations have to identify problems early on and then take action. That might sound like a criticism of current organisations, but it isn't really. You need to know what you are looking for. If you don't then you can be as well-meaning as you like but you will act too late to help someone. You will act when it 'looks' bad enough. That is too late.

And this doesn't just have to be about the highest profile stars. The patterns of behaviour will be similar and there will always be enough warning signs before things escalate really badly. Sport is going to keep pumping out players who are entertaining both on and off their fields of play, but rather than just enjoying the fun while it lasts, I would like clubs and governing bodies to act faster. Get the right people close to these sorts of individuals, to watch them and talk to them. Offer them guidance to try to avoid the escalation of their behaviour. Help them keep a perspective about who they truly are. Be able to offer them a hand of support even when their ego is pumping out an invincible persona. Just stick really close to them. In the end, it might save them, or it might not, but at least we will have tried.

Professional sport has to do far better now and in future years.

Chapter 13

I hope this book prompts readers to examine what their concept of an addict is and what they believe they need to do to get better. But that's as far as I'll go.

I'm not going to put forward definitions for you and I'm not going to suggest a particular treatment for someone. Ultimately my treatment was based around connecting with people who thought the way I did. I identified with them and some more experienced ones showed me a way to handle life differently. Without those people, I wouldn't have been able to do it on my own and, importantly, without their continual support, I wouldn't be able to keep growing as I am.

By sharing my experience, I hope that someone might identify with it and feel less alone in the world. And this is regardless of whether they have exhibited addictive behaviour patterns or not. I believe that we all struggle at various times in our lives, and this can make us act out in some form or another.

Within professional sport, some of the individuals who need help don't need to be lectured on what they are and what treatment they need; they need to connect with someone with whom they can identify. Then they will feel less alone and this will allow them to find the answers they are looking for. At some point, professional sport needs to learn from history and stop repeating the same mistakes. Laughing along with someone, and then judging and shaming them, doesn't have good consequences. There are better ways to deal with these things.

In the end, I believe we can and should help each other. It doesn't matter if you are a sports superstar or a fan in the stands; people will always benefit from feeling less alone.

***

So where have I got to now?

I have spent most of my life trying to find peace. Trying to find something to make me feel less confused about my place on the earth. Trying to find something to tell me that it all makes sense.

I have just been searching.

Through all that has happened to me, I have realised that the search is not needed. The answers were with me all along. The thing I was looking for was me and I was there the whole time. I have spent so much time searching in the past and the future, that I had missed the beauty of the now. I had missed the fact that in the now, the best version of me was right there.

My first sponsor was Roy, a wonderful man full of love and compassion. He came from football and we shared that link to professional sport. He would often cry when he shared his experiences and thoughts – not through sadness but through his passion to connect with someone else. I will always be grateful for Roy being in my life. I used to meet him for coffee, and I would be watching the clock. In my mind I had about an hour before I needed to get back to my 'important' life. I had emails to answer, tweets to write and people to remind how amazing I was. Roy would take an absolute age choosing his cake to go with his coffee. The more I twitched, the longer he took. It was like my impatience was intrinsically linked to his lack of urgency. It was unbearable at times. But as we settled at the table, he would look at me and say, 'This is what it is all about, Luke. Right now. This is the most important thing in our lives right now. This moment. Coffee and cake with a good friend.'

Like with many things on my journey, I had no idea what he meant to start with. He would say it almost every time we met. He would never really explain it in any more depth; he would just leave it with me.

Roy would often text me to say he was outside in the sun enjoying an ice cream and some sparkling water, and he just wanted to tell me how happy he was for his life and the people in it. He would thank me for being his friend. I could always imagine him crying with joy as he texted it. There was never any mention of money or status or reputation or success: it was pure.

Roy never forced me to change my attitude, he just showed me a different way and eventually I realised what he meant.

I realised that peace lies not in searching, it lies in the now. It lies not in the past and not in the future, but in the very essence of now. It lies in enjoying that coffee and cake with a friend, it lies within that moment you share with your son or daughter, it lies within observing the beauty of nature, and in sport, it lies within the beauty of that special skill on a sporting field and not in being consumed with what that might mean in the bigger picture. It lies within the stillness of a moment. Peace is there all the time; it was me who was disturbing it.

I love going to watch live sport now more than ever but not because of what results might mean for me or people I know. It is because there are moments of beauty within every contest … those moments when it feels like everything is standing still and the past and future are entirely irrelevant. Those moments when you witness extraordinary skill or bravery. It's completely magical. And those moments are in the now. Your mind is solely focused on that moment and within that lies perfect peace.

I have understood what it means to truly live in the now.

Please don't think I now live in a space that means I don't think ahead or reflect on the past. Of course I do. I love a good plan. But I am not beholden by outcomes. They don't define me. The processes define me, but I leave the outcomes to the universe and accept everything exactly as it is. This change in mindset and attitude has given me freedom from the pressures of life. I just try to live every moment as the best I can be right at that time.

And I am grateful for all the mistakes I have made. I am sorry for the pain they caused, but they have got me to where I am now. Without them, I might have never known and been searching forever. But this doesn't mean to say I have all the answers. I really don't. In fact, I have just stopped searching for the answers. I don't know what is right for other people and I don't even want to opine on that. I just know what is right for me.

And I don't live on some perfect fluffy cloud. I often get things wrong. I'm a flawed man.

Working within talent management means that I am permanently dealing with expectation. Expectation of clients, clubs, sponsors and fans. And with expectation comes disappointment, and from that can often come conflict. So I spend a lot of my working life dealing with conflict and difficult situations. That is really challenging because it can make me worry about the past and the future. And when I do, I can get in a muddle and fall out with people. I can quickly skip back to being controlling, self-obsessed and overly sensitive.

I have been through a marriage breakdown that has been incredibly difficult. I want my children to feel loved, supported and understood. I want them to feel safe in the world so that one day they can feel free to be whatever it is they want to be – without expectation or burden from me. But it's difficult. And when I don't get it right, it is always because I have slipped back into old thinking.

My family have been through an enormous amount with me. I have put them through worry and pain, and with it I have been trying to process everything with them. That hasn't been easy for any of us.

But over time, I think I am getting it wrong less and less. I know that I just have to try to be the best version of myself that I can be and leave the outcomes to sort themselves out. All I have to do is be the best father, partner, son, brother, friend, manager, business partner and ex-husband I can be. Just focus on being the best human being I can be.

When I am at my best, life feels simple and pure. I go with the flow and concentrate on the next right thing to do. When I'm not at my best, I get anxious about what's going to happen next and insecure about what people think about me. I revert back to my old self. But I have realised that there is no permanent state within this. There is no perfect. It's a journey with no end but I have a better way to live.

***

Life is really good now.

I feel like I have finally reached a place in my life where I truly understand myself. Within my work of talent management, I feel that

I can offer help to the people I work with, not just through my business experience within the sport and entertainment industries, but also through my own life experiences. I am in a position to really support young people within these environments. I know that helping others helps my own well-being, so I am in a really privileged position.

And I want to share one more thing with you because it is really relevant to my journey.

I have found my soulmate. The absolute love of my life. It is the purest love imaginable. It is love without expectation, judgement, manipulation, conditions or agenda. Love that is exactly what it should be – limitless. It is beautiful.

But the reason I share this is because this has come to me because I have changed. I became ready for that love. I became ready to understand what unconditional love truly means. It means without transaction, and to be able to give that I had to truly understand how to let go and give myself entirely to someone. How to be completely and utterly vulnerable. I wasn't capable of ever doing that previously. I was too dominated by fear and ego. But I know myself now.

In Jo, I have found my perfect partner in life. We were ready for each other.

I wish it for everyone.

***

Forgive me because I have stolen some of this from a wonderful bit of reading:

> There is no more aloneness, with that awful ache, so deep in my heart that nothing before could ever reach it. That ache is gone and never need return again. Now there is a sense of belonging, of being wanted and needed and loved. I can live my best life now.

Acknowledgements

Mum and Dad – I know I haven't been an easy son at times so thank you for constantly giving me love. The peace I have now is in part down to your unrelenting support for me.

Jo – this book wouldn't have been possible without you. I love you with every part of my being. Thank you for you.

Noel – I love you and you are still my hero.

Jude – thank you for all the love and support you gave me through some incredibly difficult times. You are a wonderful mother to Albie and Amelie, and I am forever grateful for who you are.

Lenny and everyone else I was with in The Priory – I know these aren't your real names but you know who you are. I love you all and I wish you the peace in your lives that you deserve.

Richard and the other therapists in The Priory – again, not your real names, but thank you from the bottom of my heart. You gave me compassion, time and understanding when I desperately needed it. You are truly wonderful people.